PARENTERAL
QUALITY CONTROL

ADVANCES IN PARENTERAL SCIENCES

EDITOR

JOSEPH R. ROBINSON

Center for Health Sciences
University of Wisconsin
Madison, Wisconsin

PARENTERAL
QUALITY CONTROL

Sterility, Pyrogen, Particulate, and Package Integrity Testing

MICHAEL J. AKERS

Eli Lilly and Company
Indianapolis, Indiana

MARCEL DEKKER, INC.   New York and Basel

Library of Congress Cataloging in Publication Data

Akers, Michael J.
  Parenteral quality control.

  (Advances in parenteral sciences ; 1)
  Includes bibliographies and index.
  1. Parenteral solutions--Analysis. 2. Parenteral
solutions--Standards. 3. Drug trade--Quality control.
I. Title. II. Series.
RS201.P37A54 1985   615'.19   85-7063
ISBN 0-8247-7357-8

MARCEL DEKKER, INC.
270 Madison Avenue, New York, New York 10016

Current printing (last digit):
10 9 8 7 6 5 4 3 2 1

PRINTED IN THE UNITED STATES OF AMERICA

This book is dedicated to
Mary, Scott, Ryan, and Allison

Series Introduction

The field of parenterals has seen substantial technical and scientific growth over the past two decades, with the expectation of even greater activity during the last half of the 1980s and through the 1990s. This growth is due, in part, to the expected surge in the number of very potent and sensitive peptides that are arising out of the proliferating genetic engineering programs; an expected increase in the number and type of nutritional products; and the increasing demand for expanded home health care. It is entirely appropriate, therefore, that a scientific/technical series be established not only to report on advances in this field but also to help integrate the various disciplines that impact on parenteral products.

To place the series in perspective it may be useful to provide a personal impression of the level and complexity of the parenteral field. Parenteral activities can arbitrarily be divided into (1) those devoted to making an elegant, safe and effective product, (2) the interface of that product with the route of administration, and (3) the influence of the product on the time course and biological activity of the drug in question. Naturally, all three areas are related and are not easily segregated, especially the latter two.

The technical aspects of parenterals include assurance of stability, sterility, and freedom from particulates as major concerns. These areas have received considerable attention and significant advances have been made in conventional, that is, non-sustained release parenterals. Sustained forms of parenteral products require special consideration from a preparation and quality assurance point of view.

Less well studied is the interaction of the product with the biological interface, for example, biocompatibility, local metabolism and immunological reaction. These areas require a variety of disciplines to fully understand the parenteral product—biological interface. This is a field that has been studied in an uneven manner over the years, providing a less than satisfactory data base.

The last area is the influence of the product on the time course and biological activity of the drug, the so-called bioavailability issue. In the absence of a suitable understanding of the product-biological interface, that is, point number two, it is difficult to provide a thorough mechanistic description.

Thus, there is considerable need for additional work in the area of parenterals. It is hoped that the series "Advances in Parenteral Sciences" will provide a suitable platform to record advances in this exciting field.

Joseph R. Robinson

Preface

Drug products administered by injection are characterized by three qualities possessed by no other type of pharmaceutical dosage form: sterility, freedom from pyrogenicity, and, for solutions, freedom from particulate matter. The achievement of sterile, non-pyrogenic, and particulate-free parenteral products provides a significant challenge to the ingenuity and creativity of parenteral scientists and technologists. Of equal challenge is the successful application and performance of analytical testing procedures to verify the claims of parenteral products that, indeed, they are sterile, pyrogen-free, and free from visible particulate contamination.

Regardless of the type of dosage form, quality control testing and evaluation begin with the analysis of all raw material (drug, chemical, and packaging) specifications. During the production process, quality control is vitally involved on a daily basis in the testing, checking, and monitoring of all phases of the process. Once the final product is made, it is subjected to as many tests as are necessary to ensure the potency, purity, identity, and quality of the product. Quality control testing will continue on the finished product throughout its shelf life to monitor the physical, chemical, and microbiological stability of the dosage form and its packaging system.

Finished product quality control of parenteral dosage forms requires additional tests corresponding to the unique properties of these dosage forms. *Sterility tests* evaluate the potential of the products to be contaminated with microbiological impurities. *Pyrogen tests* evaluate the capability of the product to cause an increase in the body temperature of rabbits or to cause a gel to form in the presence of *Limulus* amebocyte lysate. *Clarity tests* check for the presence of visible particulate contamination and *particulate analytical tests* go a step further to quantitate the number and size of particulate contamination. Additionally, for glass-sealed ampuls and other parenteral packaging systems, *package integrity tests* are performed to test the potential for the ingress of microbiological contamination.

Official compendial tests for sterility, pyrogens, and particulates evoke widespread controversy regarding their reliability, sensitivity, and applicability. While impressive technological advances have been made in the production of parenteral products, the testing for the quality of these products involves relatively simple procedures. One of the objectives of the book is to critique the adequacy of current methods for sterility, pyrogen, particulate, and leaker testing and to review future trends and improved technology in these areas.

The major aim of this book is to provide an educational service to individuals in industrial, hospital, and government laboratories who are involved with one or more of these specific parenteral quality control testing procedures. Much of what is learned about parenteral quality control is "on-the-job" training and experience with little or no formal education. A single, current, and comprehensive textbook totally devoted to sterility, pyrogen, particulate, and package integrity testing, as this book claims to be, could provide a useful service and fulfill a need in the learning experience of the quality control manager, hospital pharmacist, microbiologist, and laboratory technician.

The book is divided into four chapters, in the same order as the title of the book. The approach and organization of each chapter involves three basic concepts. First, a detailed description and analysis of the current United States Pharmacopeial testing procedure and requirements are presented. Next, what are the advantages and limitations of the current compendial testing procedures? Finally, what alternatives are available and what are future trends and methods with regard to the current testing procedures for parenteral quality control?

Major emphasis is placed on the practical application of testing methodology. A lesser, but appropriate, emphasis is given to the theoretical aspects of each type of quality control test procedure.

By reading and studying this book it is hoped that the reader will better learn and understand the theory and practice of parenteral quality control.

This book could not have been completed without the significant help and advice from the following individuals: Dr. Aubrey Outschoorn, Dr. Michael J. Groves, Mr. Lowell R. Lowary, Mr. Julius R. Knapp, and Dr. Joseph R. Robinson. I especially thank Dr. Kenneth E. Avis for providing me the opportunity to teach in these areas and develop some expertise to write a book on parenteral quality control. Many individuals were very responsive to requests for photographs, figures, and other information. These include Mr. John Connor (The West Co.), Mr. H. T. Shimizu (Eisai), Mr. Louis F. Brown (Cozzoli), Mr. Don Wright (Abbott), Dr. Robert Abshire (Alcon), Mr. C. Papastephanou (Squibb), Mr. William Lenzie (American McGaw), Dr. Henry F. Hammer (Pfizer), Mr. Richard Johnson (Travenol), Dr. Jeanne Baer (Burroughs-Wellcome), Dr. A. E. DeWald (Smith Kline & French), Dr. Alan Gray (Merck Sharp & Dohme), Mr. Paul Roman (Eli Lilly), and Mr. Tom Abbinett (Eli Lilly, deceased). Also, I thank the many manufacturers and publishers referenced in the text for their permission to use their figures and tables. Lastly, I certainly appreciate the excellent efforts of Mr. Kurt DeKemper for many of the photographs appearing in the book, Mr. Bill Kruse for all the artwork, and Mrs. Cyndi Lammers for typing the manuscript.

Michael J. Akers

Contents

PARENTERAL
QUALITY CONTROL

1
Sterility Testing

INTRODUCTION

Sterility, or freedom from the presence of viable microorganisms, is a strict, uncompromising requirement of an injectable dosage form. Unlike enteral administration, parenteral (Greek, *para enteron* = beside the intestine) administration of drugs avoids many of the natural protective barriers of the body. The injection of a product contaminated with living microorganisms would invite a multitude of complications to an already sick patient.

When the term "sterile" appears on the label of a parenteral product, it means that the batch or lot from which the sample originated passed the requirements of the United States Pharmacopeia (USP) sterility test. The USP sterility test provides an estimate of the probable, not actual, sterility of a lot of articles. The actual product administered to a patient itself has not been tested for sterility. The sterility test is a destructive test; thus it is impossible to test every single item for sterility. This presents a major limitation of the sterility test. Sterility is based on the results of the testing of a small number of batch samples assuming that these samples are representative of every article from the batch not tested for sterility. The question of the sample being representative of the whole will always be an uncertainty. Furthermore, another limitation of the sterility test is the finite frequency of accidental (or inadvertent) contamination of one or more samples during the performance of the testing procedures. Regardless of the perfection attempted in the attitudes and techniques involved in sterility testing, accidental contamination will occur with a given percentage of test conducted.

In light of these and other limitations of the USP sterility test, why is it still a requirement of and enforced by the Food and Drug Administration (FDA) and other regulatory agencies? The most important and obvious reason is to provide some means of end-product testing to protect the consumer from being administered a contaminated injectable product. While the sterility test does not assure sterility of every single article, it does provide the FDA as well as the manufacturer and the user with some end-point check that a representative sample of the batch does not disclose the existence of a high proportion of contaminated units in a lot or batch. End-product sterility testing also presents a reliable means of checking the sterility of a product that has been sterilized by marginal steriliza-processes such as aseptic filtration. Even if more reliable sterilization methods are used, sterility testing provides an additional means of checking that all facets of the sterilization process were achieved. For example, although steam sterilization is the most reliable sterilization process known to man, improper loading of the autoclave might prevent adequate steam penetration of some of the product containers in the batch. A statistically sound sampling procedure (again, a necessary assumption of the sterility test) will select one or more of those improperly exposed containers and the sterility test will show contamination. Nevertheless, it must be recognized, as it is by the USP, that the sterility test was not designed to ensure product sterility or sterilization process efficacy (1). It simply is a procedure used for sterility control and assurance, along with many other procedures used in manufacture to assure the sterility of a product.

This chapter will present a thorough and practical analysis of the official testing requirements for sterility, their advantages and limitations, and current adjunct processes and controls to aid in the proper performance and valid interpretation of the sterility test. Major review articles by Bowman (2), Borick and Borick (3), Beloian (4) and Outschoorn (5) were extremely helpful in the writing of this chapter.

STERILITY AND STERILITY TEST REGULATIONS

Sterility is the most important and absolutely essential characteristic of a parenteral product. Sterility means the complete absence of *all* microorganisms. It is an absolute term, that is, a product is either sterile or it is not sterile. Building sterility into a product through meticulous cleaning, filtration, and validated sterilization procedures is far preferable to the testing for sterility of a product subjected to marginal or inadequate production processes. The sterility test should never be employed as an evaluation of the sterilization process. Sterility and quality cannot be tested into a product; they can only be components of controlled processes throughout the production sequence (6). The sterility test, however, should be employed as one of several checkpoints in reaching a conclusion that the production process has removed or destroyed all living microorganisms in the product (2).

The USP chapter on injections states that preparations for injection meet the requirements under "Sterility Tests." After meeting these requirements, that is, all media vessels incubated with product sample reveal no evidence of microbial growth (turbidity), the tested product may be judged to meet the requirements of the test. If evidence for microbial growth is found, the material tested has *failed* to meet the requirements of the test for sterility. Retesting is allowed to ascertain the possibility that test failure was due to accidental contamination.

Evidence for microbial growth is determined by visual evaluation of a vessel containing the product sample in the proper volume and composition of nutrient solution. Provided that the growth conditions are optimal—proper nutrients, pH, temperature, atmosphere, sufficient incubation time, etc.—a single microbial cell will grow by geometric progression* until the number of microbial cells and their metabolic products exceeds the solubility capability of the culture medium. Manifestation of this "overgrowth" is visualized by the appearance of a cloudy or turbid solution of culture media. A noxious odor may also accompany the turbid appearance of the contaminated media. The sterility test is failed by a product that generates turbidity in a vessel of culture medium while the same lot of medium without the product sample show no appearance of turbidity.

Parenteral drug administration was a routine practice in the early 1900s. For example, insulin was discovered in 1921 and was, as it is today, administered by subcutaneous injection. Yet the first official compendial requirement of sterility testing of drugs administered by the parenteral route did not appear until 1932 in the

---

*Microbial growth may be characterized by the equation $N = 2^{gt}$, where N is the number of microbial cells, g is the number of generations or replications, and t is the time period during growth.

TABLE 1.1 Summary of Changes and Improvements in the USP Requirements for Sterility Testing

Year	USP edition	Change or improvement
1936	11th	First year sterility test appeared, applied only to sterile liquids
1942	12th	Aerobic sterility test in sterile solids and liquids Procedures for inactivation of certain preservatives
1945	13th	Fluid thioglycollate medium introduced for recovery of aerobic and anaerobic bacteria Honey medium introduced for recovery of molds and yeasts Brief description of laboratory area and training of personnel to perform sterility tests
1950	14th	Incubation temperature of FTM lowered from 37°C to 32–35°C Sabouraud liquid medium (modified) replaced honey medium
1955	15th	USP Fluid Sabouraud medium replaced the modified Sabouraud medium
1970	18th	Soybean-casein digest medium replaced Sabouraud medium Membrane filtration sterility test introduced Guidelines included for specific use of biological indicators Expanded sections on describing the area, personnel training, and techniques for performing sterility tests
1975	19th	Established separate section for membrane filtration procedures Included test procedure for large-volume solutions ($\geqslant 100$ ml)
1980	20th	Section introduced on growth promotion testing using specific indicator microorganisms Section introduced on sterility testing of prefilled disposable syringes Provide guidelines on first and second retests of suspected false positive tests

Table 1.1   (Continued)

Year	USP edition	Change or improvement
		General expansion and/or elaboration of sections of bacteriostasis, sterility testing of devices, and sterilization
		Sterilization section contains statement of $F_0 = 8$ minutes for steam-sterilized articles and D values provided for biological indicators
1985	21st	Sections on biological indicator paper strips for dry-heat sterilization, ethylene oxide sterilization, and steam sterilization
		Stricter requirements for repeating failed sterility tests
		Section on basic principles of process validation in the sterility assurance of compendial articles
		Expansion of information on sterilization by ionizing radiation and filtration
		Section on definition of a lot for sterility test purposes
		Reorganization and expansion of section on performance, observation, and interpretation of sterility test results
		Deletion of procedures for sterility testing of sutures and petrolatum gauze

British Pharmacopoeia. Sterility tests were then introduced in the 11th edition of the USP and in the sixth edition of the *National Formulary* (NF) in 1936. During the past 50 years significant changes and improvements have occurred in the official sterility test requirements, a summary of which appears in Table 1.1.

Congress passed the Federal Food, Drug, and Cosmetic (FD & C) Act in 1939 permitting the FDA to envorce the Act. The Act recognized the USP and the NF as official compendia to describe the standards of strength, quality, and purity of drugs and their dosage forms. In 1975 the two compendia were unified. In 1976 the FD & C Act was emended to recognize medical devices as entities to be included in the compendia. Thus, all drug and device products that bypass the gastrointestinal tract upon administration to a human being must pass the USP sterility test and this requirement is strictly enforced by the FDA.

Besides the USP/NF official compendia, regulations also exist for two specific groups of pharmaceuticals, the biologics (vaccines, serums, toxins, antitoxins, and blood products) and the antibiotics. Sterility tests for biologics and antibiotics are described under Title 21 of the Code of Federal Regulations (7).

SAMPLING FOR STERILITY TESTING

In pharmaceutical manufacture, the sterility of a parenteral product lot is checked by a statistically valid sampling procedure. After years of experience, most manufacturers of parenteral products will sterility test 10 to 20 units of product per lot. The number of units sampled depends on the number of units in the batch, the volume of liquid per container, the method of sterilization, the use of a biological indicator system, and the good manufacturing practice requirements of the regulatory agency for the particular product. For example, if the batch size is greater than 200 articles, a minimum of 20 units are sampled. If the final batch size is between 20 and 200 articles then not fewer than 10% of the articles are sterility tested although there are minimum requirements for sterility testing of biologics. For large-volume parenteral (LVP) products (volume $\geq$100 ml per container), at least 10 containers are sampled. Only 10 test units are sampled for products sterilized by steam under pressure. If a product is sterilized by methods other than steam under pressure, then 20 units are sampled for sterility testing. However, if a biological indicator was used in the product batch, then only 10 test units are sampled for testing. Public Health Service and Antibiotic regulations require 20 final containers from each filling operation. Sampling requirements as specified in the USP sterility tests are summarized in Table 1.2.

Correct statistical sampling represents a difficult, yet vital, aspect of sterility testing. Realizing that the parenteral product being used by the patient has of itself not been tested for sterility it is absolutely essential that the sampling procedure be as valid and representative of the whole batch as possible. Realistically, this presents an impossible principle to prove.

Pharmaceutical quality control departments employ sampling plans called *acceptance sampling* for many quality control testing procedures that are not amenable to 100% final testing. Acceptance sampling in sterility testing is based on the establishment of *operating characteristic curves*, which are plots of probability versus percent contamination. Operating characteristic (OC) curves for sample sizes of 10 and 20 units are shown in Figures 1.1 and 1.2, respectively (8). These curves are drawn from a series of govern-

TABLE 1.2 Minimum Number of Units Required per Medium for Performance of the USP Sterility Test as a Function of Volume per Test Unit (Quantities for Liquid Articles)

Container content (ml)	Minimum volume taken from each container for each medium	Minimum volume of each medium		Number of containers per medium
		Used for direct transfer of volume taken from each container (ml)	Used for membrane or half membrane representing total volume from the appropriate number of containers (ml)	
Less than 10[a]	1 ml, or entire contents if less than 1 ml	15	100	20 (40 if each does not contain sufficient volume for both media)
10 to less than 50[a]	50 ml	40	100	20
50 to less than 100[a]	10 ml	80	100	20
50 to less than 100, intended for intravenous administration[b]	Entire contents	--	100	10
100 to 500[a]	Entire contents	--	100	10
Over 500[a]	500 ml	--	100	10

[a]Intended for multiple dose or non-intravenous use.
[b]Intended for single dose or intravenous use.

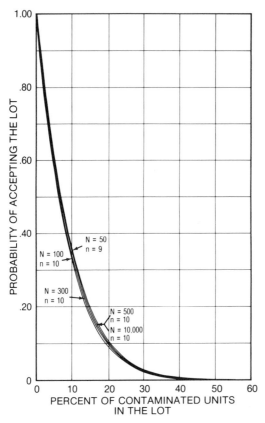

FIGURE 1.1 Operating characteristic curves for a sample size of
10 units. n = sample size; N = lot size. (From Ref. 8.)

ment-sponsored sampling plans called MIL-STD-414 (9). The shape
of the curve depends on five criteria:

1. An acceptable quality level (AQL), which is the highest
    percentage of defective (non-sterile) units that is acceptable
2. An unacceptable quality level (UQL), which is the percentage
    of non-sterile units for which there is a low probability of
    acceptance.
3. The alpha (α) factor, which is the probability of rejecting
    a good (sterile) batch.

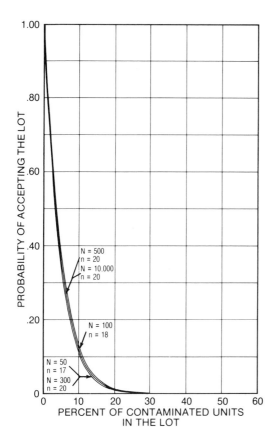

FIGURE 1.2 Operating characteristic curves for a sample size of 20 units. n = sample size; N = lot size. (From Ref. 8.)

4. The beta (β) error, which is the probability of accepting a bad (non-sterile) batch
5. The sample size

With all criteria (1) through (5) being constant, the slope of the OC curve will become steeper as the sample size is increased. Similarly, with the criteria being constant, the slope of the curve will become steeper as the AQL is decreased, or as the UQL is decreased. An example of an OC curve for sampling plans at AQL = 1% for different sample sizes is seen in Figure 1.3 (10). At a given

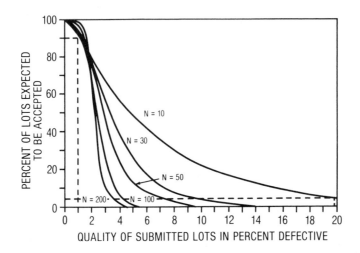

FIGURE 1.3 Operating characteristic curve for sampling plans at an acceptable quality level of 1% for different sample sizes N. (From Ref. 10.)

AQL level, the larger the sample size the greater is the probability of accepting a sterile lot and rejecting a non-sterile lot. Each pharmaceutical manufacturer for each type of parenteral product assumes a given AQL or rate of contamination, thus fixing the point of reference on the abscissa of the OC curve.

Sampling plans and concomitant OC curves are prepared on the assumption that the samples are selected at random. By random sampling, it is inferred that any one of the remaining uninspected units of the same lot of product has an equal chance of being selected (11). This is not always easily accomplished. Random sampling often is inconvenient and may not be appreciated by production workers responsible for many other important duties during the production process. Random samples are optimally selected every kth unit where k = the total units in the batch per the number of samples required. For example, if the batch size of an aseptically filled product is 10,000 units and 20 samples are required for the sterility test, then samples are taken every 500 units including the first and last unit filled.

Additional discussion of sampling with regard to its limiting the interpretation of the results of the sterility test is presented later in this chapter, in the section "Limitations of the USP/NF Referee Sterility Test."

A major consideration in sampling for sterility testing is proper treatment of the package system in order to prevent contamination of the sample when it is taken out of the package for testing. For example, parenteral products packaged in ampuls, vials, or bottles must be aseptically sampled using sterile materials and aseptic techniques. The neck of the ampul or the surface of the rubber closure must be disinfected with a liquid disinfectant solution before breaking the ampul or penetrating the closure with a needle. Special procedures must be implemented to sample products contained in aluminum foil, paper, or plastic outer bags. For example, bulk solid chemicals sterilized by ethylene oxide prior to aseptic compounding are contained in gas-permeable paper or plastic bags. The chemicals must be sampled by tearing open the package, which is not easy to do because of the potential for accidental contamination. Sutures are contained in glass or aluminum-foil enclosures which must be disinfected before the product is removed. Sampling of devices without contaminating the sample also is a very difficult procedure to accomplish. Although the package may be designed to maintain the sterility of the product indefinitely, it is obviously of no value if the inner contents cannot be removed without contaminating the product and interfering with the performance of certain essential tests (3).

CULTURE MEDIA

The USP describes two primary types of culture media to be used in the sterility testing of parenteral products. One type is called Fluid Thioglycollate Medium (FTM), which was introduced by Brewer (12) in 1949. The formulation ingredients of FTM and their basic purpose in the medium are listed below:

1.	L-cysteine	0.5 g	Antioxidant
2.	Agar, granulated	0.75 g	Nutrient and viscosity-inducer
3.	Sodium chloride	2.5 g	Isotonic agent
4.	Dextrose	5.5 g	Nutrient
5.	Yeast extract	5.0 g	Nutrient
6.	Pancreatic digest of casein	15.0 g	Nutrient
7.	Sodium thioglycollate or thioglycollic acid	0.5 g 0.3 ml	Antioxidant
8.	Resazurin sodium solution (1:1000)	1.0 ml	Oxidation indicator
9.	Water pH after sterilization	QS 1000 ml 7.1 ± 0.2	

FTM provides both aerobic and anaerobic environments within the same medium. Thioglycollate and L-cysteine are antioxidants or reducing agents that maintain anaerobiasis in the lower levels of the culture tube. FTM solution has a two-color appearance. The pinkish color of the top part of the solution is indicative of the presence of resazurin sodium, an oxygen-sensitive indicator. The pink color should consume no more than one-third of the medium volume. Because of the need for two environments in the same test tube or container, the ratio of surface to medium depth is very important. To provide adequate depth for oxygen penetration, a 15-ml volume of FTM must be contained in a test tube of the dimensions 20 × 150 mm. A 40-ml volume of FTM is to be contained in 25 × 200 mm test tubes, and 75-100 ml FTM in 38 × 200 mm test tubes.

Devices containing tubes with small lumina are sterility tested using an alternate thioglycollate medium in which the agar and resazurin sodium are deleted. The same medium is used for turbid or viscous parenterals. Without the agar the medium will not interfere with the viscosity of the product or be as resistant in filling small lumina. Since the medium will be turbid, the presence of a color indicator would not be seen anyway. For oily products, FTM is slightly modified by the addition of 1 ml Polysorbate 80 to 1 liter of the media. Polysorbate 80 serves as an emulsifying agent to permit adequate dispersal of a lipophilic product in a hydrophilic growth medium.

FTM is an excellent medium for the detection of bacterial contamination. Thioglycollate also has the advantage of neutralizing the bacteriostatic properties of the mercurial preservatives. One disadvantage of FTM is that it will not support the growth of *Bacillus subtilis* spores entrapped in solids or material that locates itself in the anaerobic lower portion of the medium (13). *B. subtilis* spores require an environment of high surface tension for normal growth.

The other primary USP/NF culture medium for the sterility testing of parenterals is called Soybean-Casein Digest (SCD) or Trypticase Soy Broth (TSB) medium. The formulation ingredients and their purpose in TSB are:

1.	Pancreatic digest of casein	17.0 g	Nutrient
2.	Papaic digest of soybean meal	3.0 g	Nutrient
3.	Sodium chloride	5.0 g	Isotonic agent
4	Dibasic potassium phosphate	2.5 g	Buffer
5.	Dextrose	2.5 g	Nutrient
6.	Water	QS 1000 ml	
	pH after sterilization	7.3 ± 0.2	

TSB has a slightly higher pH (7.3 ± 0.2) than does FTM (7.1 ±
0.2). TSB replaced Sabouraud medium in the 19th edition of the
USP (1970) because TSB was found from experience to be a better
medium. It possesses a higher pH and, thus, was considered a
better nutrient for fungal contaminants (14). Fluid Sabouraud,
designed to inhibit certain bacteria, was successful in promoting
the growth of molds, fungi, and other saprophytes requiring high
dextrose content and low pH. TSB, however, promotes growth of
fungi and bacteria, and is also considered a better medium for
slow-growing aerobic microorganisms than FTM.

Other media have been proposed to replace or be substituted for
FTM and/or TSB. Abdou (15) found that a dithionite-thioglycollate
broth and a peptone liver digest medium were superior to FTM and
TSB in growing various strains of bacteria, yeasts, and molds.
Concentrated Brain Heart Infusion Broth has been suggested as an
alternative to FTM and TSB when large-volume parenterals are directly inoculated with culture medium. Table 1.3 lists the formulas
of eleven media and reagents potentially used in the sterility testing of parenteral products. While these and other media might be
appropriate for certain products or situations, it is highly unlikely
that TSB or FTM will be replaced as official USP sterility test media.

Culture media may be purchased in either the dehydrated state
or the ready-to-use fluid state. Dehydrated media are less expensive and have a longer shelf-life. Strict adherence to the expira-
tion date on the label of pre-mixed culture media tubes must be
obeyed, provided that the proper storage conditions (usually
refrigeration) have been met.

Preparation of sterile fluid culture media from dehydrated media
is a relatively simple process. The label of each container of medium describes the procedure for preparation. Basically, the procedure involves (a) weighing the appropriate amount of medium per
liter of fluid desired, (b) adding water to the compounding vessel
to the desired volume, (c) slowly adding the culture medium while
stirring the solution, (d) applying heat and stirring until the medium is completely dissolved, and (e) sterilizing the medium in bulk
or after filling into test tubes or other containers by steam heat
under pressure by a validated sterilization cycle. Before discard-
ing culture media, they must be again sterilized by steam under
pressure before pouring the fluid into a drainage system and
washing the containers.

When membrane filtration is used for the sterility test, a diluting
fluid must be used to rinse the filtration assembly in order to ensure that no microbial cells remain anywhere but on the filter surface. The diluting fluid may also be used to dissolve a sterile solid
prior to filtration. Some examples of diluting fluid formulas are

TABLE 1.3 Media and Reagents Potentially Used in Performing the USP/NF Sterility Tests[a]

USP fluid thioglycollate (thio) medium. Use BBL 11260 or Difco 0256.

Trypticase Peptone (BBL) or Bacto-Casitone (Difco)	15.0 g
L-Cysteine	0.5 g
Dextrose (anhydrous)	5.0 g
Yeast extract	5.0 g
Sodium chloride	2.5 g
Sodium thioglycollate	0.5 g
Resazurin (1:1000)	1.0 ml
Agar	0.75 g
Distilled water	1.0 liter
Final ph 7.1	

USP soybean-casein digest medium. Use Trypticase Soy Broth (BBL 11768) or Tryptic Soy Broth (Difco 0370).

Trypticase Peptone (BBL) or Bacto-Tryptone (Difco)	17.0 g
Phytone Peptone (BBL) or Bacto-Soytone (Difco)	3.0 g
Sodium chloride	5.0 g
Dipotassium phosphate	2.5 g
Dextrose	2.5 g
Distilled water	1.0 liter
Final pH 7.3	

Polysorbate 80. A suitable grade is TWEEN 80, available from Atlas Chemicals Division, ICI Americas Inc.

Brain heart infusion. Use BBL 11059 or Difco 0037.

Calf brain, infusion from	200.0 g
Beef heart, infusion from	250.0 g
Gelysate Peptone (BBL) or Proteose Peptone (Difco)	10.0 g
Sodium chloride	5.0 g
Disodium phosphate	2.5 g
Dextrose	2.0 g
Distilled water	1.0 liter
Final pH 7.4	

TABLE 1.3 (Continued)

Sporulating agar medium. Use AK Agar No. 2
(Sporulating Agar) (BBL 10912) or Sporulating
Agar (Difco 0582).

Gelysate Peptone (BBL) or Bacto-Peptone (Difco)	6.0 g
Trypticase Peptone (BBL) or Bacto-Casitone (Difco)	4.0 g
Yeast extract	3.0 g
Beef extract	1.5 g
Dextrose	1.0 g
Agar	15.0 g
Manganous sulfate	0.3 g
Distilled water	1.0 liter
Final pH 6.5	

Saline TS, Sterile (USP)

Sodium chloride	9.0 g
Distilled water	1.0 liter

Sabouraud dextrose agar medium. Use BBL 11584
or Difco 0109.

Dextrose	40.0 g
Polypeptone (BBL) or Neopeptone (Difco)	10.0 g
Agar	15.0 g
Distilled water	1.0 liter
Final pH 5.6	

USP soybean-casein digest agar medium. Use Trypticase Soy Agar (BBL 11043) or Tryptic Soy Agar (Difco 0369).

Trypticase Peptone (BBL) or Bacto-Tryptone (Difco)	15.0 g
Phytone Peptone (BBL) or Bacto-Soytone (Difco)	5.0 g
Sodium chloride	5.0 g
Agar	15.0 g
Distilled water	1.0 liter
Final pH 7.3	

Fluid Sabouraud Medium. Use Sabouraud Liquid
Medium (Difco 0382).

Dextrose	20.0 g
Polypeptone Peptone (BBL) or Neopeptone (Difco)	10.0 g
Distilled water	1.0 liter
Final pH 5.7	

TABLE 1.3   (Continued)

USP antibiotic (agar) medium 1.   Use BBL 10937
or Difco 0263.

Gelysate Peptone (BBL) or Bacto-Peptone (Difco)	6.0 g
Trypticase Peptone (BBL) or Bacto-Casitone (Difco)	4.0 g
Yeast extract	3.0 g
Beef extract	1.5 g
Dextrose	1.0 g
Agar	15.0 g
Distilled water	1.0 liter
Final pH 6.6	

Potato dextrose agar medium

Potato agar	15.0 g
Glucose	20.0 g
Distilled water q.s.	1.0 liter
pH 5.6 ± 0.2	

---

[a]Sterilize in an autoclave at 121°C (15 lb pressure) for 15
minutes unless otherwise indicated. If commercial preparations
are not available, equivalent preparations may be used.

TABLE 1.4 Formulations of Various Diluting Fluids Used With
the Membrane Filtration Test Method

Diluting fluid A	
Peptic digest of animal tissue	1.0 g
Distilled water	1.0 liter
(pH 7.1 ± 0.2)	
Diluting fluid D	
Peptic digest of animal tissue	1.0 g
Polysorbate 80	1.0 ml
Distilled water	1.0 liter
(pH 7.1 ± 0.2)	
Diluting fluid A modified	
Peptic digest of animal tissue	1.0 g
Ascorbic acid	10.0 g
Distilled water	1.0 liter

TABLE 1.4 (Continued)

Diluting fluid E

Isopropyl myristate	100.0 ml
(Water extract pH not less than 6.5)	

Medium K

Peptic digest of animal tissue	5.0 g
Beef extract	3.0 g
Polysorbate 80	10.0 g
Distilled water	q.s. 1.0 liter
(pH 6.9 ± 0.2)	

---

listed in Table 1.4. Diluting fluids are intended to minimize the destruction of small populations of vegetative cells during the pooling, solubilizing, and filtering of sterile pharmaceutical products (16).

TIME AND TEMPERATURE OF INCUBATION

No ideal incubation time and temperature condition exists for the harvesting of all microorganisms. Most organisms grow more rapidly at 37°C than at lower temperatures. However, a temperature of about 23°C may reveal the presence of some organisms that might remain undetected if incubations were done at higher temperatures (17). Pittman and Feeley (18) demonstrated that temperatures of 22°C and 30°C were more favorable for the recovery of yeasts and fungi in FTM than a temperature of 35°C. The Division of Biologics Standards of the National Institutes of Health discovered that a pseudomonad contaminant in plasma grew in FTM at 25°C, but was killed at 35°C (2). As a result of this finding, the incubation temperature range of FTM was lowered from 32–35°C to 30–35°C as required by the USP/NF (20th edition) and 30–32°C specifically required by the Division of Biologics.

The current time and temperature incubation requirements of the USP sterility test are found in Table 1.5. Incubation in TSB is accomplished at 20–25°C because of favorable growth of fungal and slow-growing aerobic contaminants at this temperature range. The time of incubation for sterility testing by membrane filtration is seven days, less than that for the direct transfer method, because of the concentrative nature of the filtration technique.

The incubation time requirements of the sterility test must be of sufficient length to account for the variable lag time characteristic

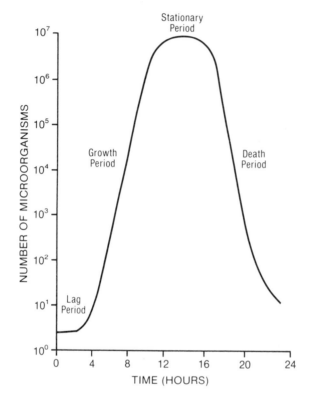

FIGURE 1.4 Typical growth and death cycle for bacteria.

of the growth curve of most microbial forms. A typical growth
cycle for bacteria is seen in Figure 1.4. At the beginning of the
cycle, corresponding to the time at which the test sample is combined with the culture medium, there exists a lag time phase. The
length of this lag time depends on the rapidity of the microbial cell
to adapt to its "new" environment. Usually the lag phase lasts no
longer than a few hours, but the possibility is always present that
a resistant spore form, a slow-growing contaminant or a microorganism with an extra long lag phase owing to damage caused in the
sterilization process may be part of the test sample. Sufficient
incubation time must be allowed for the microbial form to overcome
its own resistance to grow in the FTM or TSB environment. However, once the lag phase is completed, the growth phase is ex-
ponential. Most contaminated samples will show evidence of con-

tamination within 24 to 48 hours due to the meteoric growth of microorganisms.

With the direct transfer method it is possible that a physiochemical incompatibility between the product inoculum and the culture medium might exist, resulting in a precipitate or turbid reaction not indicative of microbial growth. Should this occur, the appropriate action to take is to transfer an aliquot of the suspension to fresh culture medium between the third and seventh day after the test was started and incubate both the original and the new media for a total of, but not less than, 14 days. Thus, in all cases the original vessels would be held for 14 days. If the transfer were made on the fourth day, the transfer vessels would be held for 10 days. Likewise, if the transfer were made on the seventh day, the vessels would be held for seven days.

Incubation time and temperature requirements of sterility tests conducted under the auspices of various authorities are basically similar to those of the USP presented in Table 1.5. The importance of time of sampling in hospital I. V. admixture sterility testing was discovered by DeChant et al. (19). They found that no more than one hour should transpire between preparation of intravenous admixtures and sampling of the admixture for conducting a sterility test. If longer time periods are permitted, microorganisms, if in-

TABLE 1.5 Time and Temperature Incubation Requirements of the USP Sterility Test

Medium	Test procedure	Time (days)[a]	Temperature(°C)
FTM	Direct transfer	14	30−35
	Membrane filtration ⩽100 ml	7	30−35
	Membrane filtration ⩾100 ml	7	30−35
TSB	Direct transfer	14	20−25
	Membrane filtration ⩽100 ml	7	20−25
	Membrane filtration ⩾100 ml	7	20−25

[a]Time is the minimum number of incubation days. Additional incubation time may be required if the nature of the product is conducive to produce a "slow-growing" contaminant.

troduced during the admixture preparation period, may be inhibited
from reproducing because of bactericidal activity of certain I. V.
solutions such as dextrose 5% in water.

STERILITY TEST METHODS

The USP specifies two basic methods for performing sterility tests—
the direct transfer or direct inoculation method and the membrane
filtration method, with a statement that the latter, where feasible,
is the method of choice. In fact, in some cases, membrane filtration may be the only possible choice. Suggested standard operating procedures for performing both methods are given at the end
of this book as Appendices I and II.

Direct Transfer Method

The direct transfer (DT) method is the more traditional sterility
test method. Basically, the DT method involves three steps:

1. Aseptically opening each sample container from a recently
   sterilized batch of product
2. Using a sterile syringe and needle to withdraw the required
   volume of sample for both media from the container
3. Injecting one-half of the required volume of sample into
   a test tube containing the required volume of FTM and the
   other half volume of sample into a second test tube containing the required volume of TSB

The DT method is simple in theory, but difficult in practice.
The technician performing the DT test must have excellent physical dexterity and the proper mental attitude about the concern
for maintaining asepsis. The demand for repetition in opening
containers, sampling, transferring, and mixing can potentially
cause fatigue and boredom with a subsequent deterioration in operator technique and concern. As this occurs, the incidence of accidental product sterility test contamination will increase.

The USP requires a minimum volume of sample per container
volume to be transferred to a minimum volume of each culture medium. Table 1.6 lists these volume requirements. The sample volume must be a sufficient representation of the entire container
volume and the volume of medium must be sufficient to promote and
expedite microbial growth, if present. Adequate mixing between
the sample inoculum and the culture medium must take place to
maximize interaction and facilitate microbial growth.

TABLE 1.6 Volume Requirements of the Direct Transfer Sterility Test

Container content (ml)	Minimum volume of product (ml)	Minimum volume of medium (ml)
10 or less	1 (or total content if less than 1 ml)	15
10–50	5	40
50–100	10	80
100–500	Total content	100
>500	500	100

Membrane Filtration Method

The membrane filtration (MF) sterility test became official in the 18th edition of the USP in 1970. It has since become the more popular and widely used method over the DT method and, when feasible for pharmacopeial articles, should be preferred. Specific application of the MF sterility test method has been the subject of many publications, e.g., the sterility testing of antibiotics (16), insulin (20), and large-volume parenterals (21).

The successful employment of this technique requires more skill and knowledge than that required for the DT method. Five basic steps are involved in the use of the MF sterility test method:

1. The filter unit (Figure 1.5) must be properly assembled and sterilized prior to use.
2. The contents of the prescribed number of units are transferred to the filter assembly under strict aseptic conditions.
3. The contents are filtered with the aid of a vacuum or pressure differential system.
4. The membrane is removed aseptically and cut in half.*
5. One-half of the membrane is placed in a suitable volume (usually 100 ml) of FTM and the other membrane half is placed in an equal volume of TSB.

---

*The USP (21st edition) gives the option of using two "whole" membranes, one for each medium, or cutting a single membrane. However, for antibiotics the CFR requires the cutting of a single membrane only.

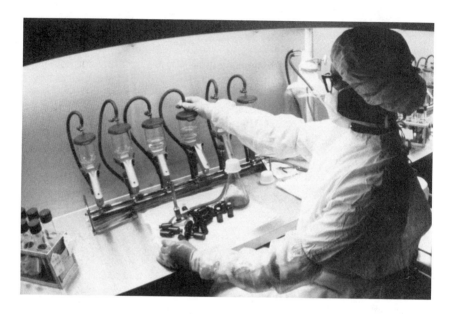

FIGURE 1.5 Set-up membrane filtration sterility test apparatus. (Courtesy of Eli Lilly and Co., Indianapolis, Indiana.)

The membrane used usually is a 0.45–0.22 micrometer porosity filter with a diameter of 47 mm and can accommodate a flow rate of 55 to 75 ml of water per minute at a pressure of 70 cm of mercury. The entire assembled unit is sterilized either by steam under pressure or by ethylene oxide. Membranes may be sterilized separately by steam under pressure or ethylene oxide; if the article to be tested is an oil, the membrane is sterilized separately in order that it may be thoroughly dried. The filter unit is then assembled under aseptic conditions.

The cleaning, assembly, sterilization, and final connections involved in the preparation of the membrane filtration equipment are described in Appendix III. Complete description and application of membrane sterility test methods for antibiotics, non-antibiotics, and ophthalmics may be studied using the Millipore Application Manual AM201, Millipore Corp., Bedford, MA 01730.

The MF method offers at least four advantages over the use of the DT method. They are:

1. The antimicrobial agent and other antimicrobial solutes in the product sample can be eliminated by filtration prior to

transferring the filter into test tubes of media, thereby minimizing the incidence of false negative test results.

2. The entire contents of containers can be tested, providing a real advantage in the sterility testing of large-volume parenterals and increasing the ability to detect contamination of product lots containing very few contaminated units.
3. Low-level contamination can be concentrated on the membrane by filtering large volumes of product.
4. Organisms present in an oleaginous product can be separated from the product during filtration and cultured in a more desirable aqueous medium.

Conversely, the MF method presents three major disadvantages when compared to the DT method:

1. There exists a higher probability of inadvertent contamination in manual operations because of the need for greater operator skill and better environmental control in disassembling the filtration unit and removing, cutting, and transferring the membrane.
2. The method is unable to differentiate the extent of contamination between units, if present, because all product concontents are combined and filtered through a single filter and cultured in single test tubes. Also, if accidental contamination has occurred, rather than this being detected in one or more vessels of the DT method, it manifests itself in the only container used per culture medium.
3. Sterilization cycles used to prepare equipment for the MF test must be validated to insure sterility of the testing equipment.

Interpretation of Results

No visible evidence of microbial growth in a culture medium test tube, after subjecting the sample and medium to the correct procedures and conditions of the USP sterility test, may be interpreted that the sample representing the lot is absent of intrinsic contamination. Such interpretation must be made by those having appropriate formal training in microbiology and having knowledge of several basic areas involved in quality control sterility tests:

1. Industrial sterilization methods and their limitations
2. Aseptic processing
3. Statistical concepts involved in sampling lots for representative articles
4. Environmental control procedures used in the test facility

If microbial growth is found or if the sterility test is judged to be invalid because of incorrect or inadequate testing environment, then the test must be repeated. The USP requires several aspects of the production and control records to be reviewed before repeating the test:

1. Monitoring records of the validated sterilization cycle applicable to the product
2. Sterility test history of the product for both finished and in-process samples
3. Sterilization records of supporting equipment, containers/closures, and sterile components, if any
4. Environmental control data—media fills, exposure plates, filtration records, sanitizing records, microbial monitoring records of operators, gowns, gloves, and garbing practices

If the above review fails to provide an explanation for the test failure, the current microbial profile of the product, i.e., what specific microorganisms were found in the failed test, should be checked against the known historical profile of the product to see if any new contamination has occurred. Also, checks should be done to ascertain any changes in sources of product components and/or in-process procedures.

If all these review procedures fail to reveal the cause of microbial growth in the First Stage sterility test, the test will be repeated as a Second Stage test. If a cause was found to invalidate the original test, the test will be repeated as a First Stage test. A Second Stage test usually includes double the number of test samples although the USP does not specify the particular number of specimens. A repeat First Stage test uses the same number of test samples. The minimum volumes tested from each specimen, the media, and the incubation periods remain the same as those used for the initial test.

If no microbial growth is found in the Second Stage, and the documented review of appropriate records and product details does not support the possibility of intrinsic contamination, the lot passes the requirements of the test for sterility. However, if growth is found again, the lot fails to meet the requirements of the test. The only way the Second Stage test can be repeated is for the test to be judged invalid for reasons and evidence as discussed above.

STERILITY TESTING OF DIFFERENT STERILE PRODUCTS

The USP describes the sterility test procedures to be followed for all types of sterile products excluding human biologics, human antibiotics, and veterinary biologics, to which Federal regulations (9CFR113.26) apply. Test procedures for the direct transfer to test media are given for the following six types of products:

1. Liquids
2. Ointments and oils insoluble in isopropyl myristate
3. Solids
4. Purified cotton, gauze, surgical dressings, sutures, and related articles
5. Sterilized devices
6. Prefilled disposable syringes

Test procedures for using the MF technique are specified for the following four types of products:

1. Liquids miscible with aqueous vehicles
2. Liquids immiscible with aqueous vehicles, less than 100 ml per container
3. Ointments and oils soluble in isopropyl myristate
4. Devices

For complete descriptions of these test procedures, please refer to the appropriate section of the USP. In the following discussion, each test procedure will be summarized with additional information not found in the USP description for the enhancement of the reader's understanding and appreciation of the procedure.

1. Direct transfer of liquids to test media

    Summary of procedure: A sterile pipet or syringe and needle is used to transfer aseptically the specified volume of liquid from each test container to a vessel of culture medium. The combination is mixed, then incubated for at least 14 days. The USP describes a further procedure, previously covered in this chapter (page 19) for transferring inoculated media when they have been rendered turbid by the test sample.

    Commentary: The risk of inadvertent contamination is at its greatest during this process. *Strict aseptic technique* must be practiced in order to minimize this risk. Also, it must be realized that a finite probability exists that the pipet or syringe and needle may themselves not be sterile.
    The USP cautions against excessive mixing of the test sample and the medium. This is especially true for FTM because of the need to preserve the efficacy of the thioglycollate antioxidant, which maintains anaerobiasis in the upper part of the vessel.

At least 14 days are required to ensure that any microbial contaminants, if present, have been given sufficient time to adapt to the FTM or TSB environment and begin to thrive and reproduce.

2. Direct transfer of ointments and oils to test media

Summary of procedure: 100 mg from each of 10 containers are aseptically transferred to a flask containing 100 ml of a sterile aqueous vehicle. 10 ml of this mixture is then mixed with 80 ml of FTM and incubated for not less than 14 days. The entire process described above is repeated with another 10 containers using TSB as the medium.

Commentary: Two key facets of this procedure are: (a) employing strict aseptic technique in the *two* transfer processes for each medium, and (b) choosing the correct dispersing agent in the aqueous vehicle that both adequately disperses the oil or ointment homogeneously in the vehicle and, in the concentration used, has no antimicrobial capacity in and of itself. The most commonly used dispersing agents are surface active agents such as Polysorbate 80 and Triton X-100 dissolved in water. Some feel, however, that Triton X-100 exerts an antimicrobial effect.

3. Direct transfer of solids to test media

Summary of procedure: The sterile solid (300 mg or the entire mass if less than 300 mg), either as is or reconstituted as a solution or suspension with a sterile diluent, is transferred to not less than 40 ml of FTM. This is repeated for TSB. The number of containers per medium usually is 20. The incubation time is again not less than 14 days.

Commentary: Most sterility testing facilities prefer reconstituting the dry sterile solid with sterile water for injection. The chance of accidental contamination is greatly enhanced because of the extra manipulations involved in reconstituting and then withdrawing the fluid sample for transfer. The adherence to strict aseptic technique cannot be overemphasized.

4. Direct transfer of purified cotton, gauze, surgical dressings, sutures, and related articles to test media

Summary of procedure: The material is transferred directly to culture media using sterile instruments such as sterile forceps and sterile scissors. Sutures are contained in glass or aluminum foil enclosures. Immerse the enclosure for three hours or more in a suitable antimicrobial solution containing a dye. The enclosure is then removed with sterile forceps and viewed for evidence of leakage. If no leakage has oc- curred, open the enclosures aseptically and transfer the sutures to containers of FTM and TSB with sterile forceps. For petrolatum gauze, the entire contents of a single package is transferred to 300 ml of specially prepared and sterilized FTM solution at a temperature of 52°C. The mixture is shaken and cooled until the petrolatum forms a solid seal over the medium surface. The seal is broken, then the medium is incubated for not less than 7 days at 20−25°C. After this initial incubation, the medium is shaken again and 0.5 ml of the mixture is transferred aseptically to 15 ml of culture medium where incubation is done again at 30−35°C for not less than seven days. Media and incubation condi- tions are identical to those already described.

Commentary: If the entire article is too large to be trans- ferred intact to culture media, a suitable portion or the in- nermost part of the article is cut out and assumed to be representative of the entire article. The rationale for select- ing the innermost part is the fact that this part is the most difficult area for steam or gas to penetrate during terminal sterilization. The antimicrobial solution used is either aqueous glutaraldehyde or alcoholic formaldehyde. The min- imum time of three hours is necessary to assure destruction of microbial spores on the package. The dye, either crystal violet or methylene blue, is used to detect an improper or weak seal which, if present, would allow penetration of the chemosterilizer into the container and lead to a false sterility test result (3). For petrolatum gauze, the specially pre- pared FTM contains more agar and the addition of gelatin to produce a more viscous medium for accommodating the petrolatum semi-solid material.

5. Direct transfer of sterilized devices to test media

Summary of procedure: The size and geometry of the device determine the type of sterility test procedure. For devices that are small enough, such as small syringes, small pipets and pipet tips, small in-line filters, needles, and the like, the entire device is immersed in not more than 1000 ml of both FTM and TSB. Fluid administration devices whose fluid pathway is claimed to be sterile are flushed with FTM and TSB, employing 20 devices per medium. The medium is

emptied from the lumen, combined with additional medium
(not less than 100 ml) and incubated for 14 days. In some
systems having very small lumens, FTM is replaced with alternative thioglycollate medium. In the case of unwieldy devices too large to too complex in shape for the device to be
sterility tested intact, the part of the article considered to
be the most difficult to sterilize is removed and placed in not
more than 1000 ml of culture medium. An example would be
a large plastic syringe dispenser unit, such as that shown in
Figure 1.6. The tubing and stopcock section is detached
from the syringe and immersed in culture media. When the
device or specimen has antimicrobial effects, it must be
rinsed with a suitable fluid which is then tested by
membrane filtration.

Commentary: A cylindrical glass culture vessel equipped
with a vented nylon closure has been developed as a sterility
test vessel for sterile devices of various sizes and shapes
(22). The vessel is easy to charge with medium and to

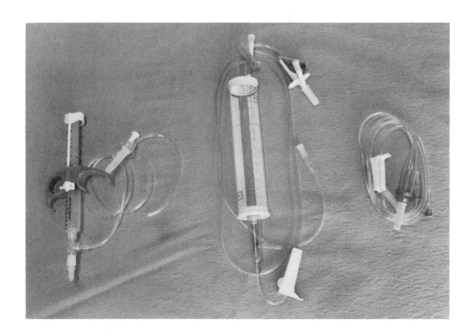

FIGURE 1.6 Example of a large plastic syringe dispenser unit.

sterilize, has a wide opening for entry of large devices, and is less likely to allow contamination entering during storage, inoculation, and incubation.

6. Direct transfer of empty or prefilled syringes to test media

    Summary of procedure: The syringe product is treated like a vial or ampul in performing the sterility test. A needle is aseptically attached, if not already part of the set, to transfer the contents to vessels of culture media. After the product has been transferred, or where the syringe assembly is empty, sterile media is flushed through each syringe and/or the lumen of each needle and incubated. Each needle itself, if part of the product, is immersed in media to demonstrate sterility of the outer part of the needle.

    Commentary: The frequency of use of prefilled disposable syringes has increased significantly in recent years. In many instances, syringes are prefilled in hospital pharmacies. Therefore, hospital pharmacists must be trained in performing sterility tests and maintaining proper aseptic techniques in performing the tests. Aseptic technique is also especially important in cases where a needle must be attached later to the prefilled syringe.

The next five procedures discuss the application of the membrane filtration sterility test involving different sterile products:

1. Membrane filtration of liquids miscible with aqueous vehicles

    Summary of procedure: At least 20 containers of product are used. Sufficient volumes required for both media are transferred aseptically into the membrane filter funnel. Vacuum or pressure is applied and the solution is filtered. The membrane is removed aseptically and cut in half; one half is placed in 100 ml of FTM while the other half is placed in 100 ml of TSB. Incubation is carried out for not less than 7 days.
    For large-volume parenteral (LVP) solutions, 50 ml to less than 100 ml for I. V. use, or between 100 ml and 500 ml, the entire contents of 10 containers are aseptically transferred and filtered through each of two filter assemblies or, if only one filter assembly is used, then 20 containers are emptied. For LVP solutions of volumes greater than 500 ml, at least 500 ml are transferred from each of 10 containers

through each of two filter assemblies, or from each of 20 containers if one filter assembly is used. Then the membrane is removed using sterile forceps, cut in half with sterile scissors, and the halves aseptically added to 100 ml of FTM and TSB, respectively.

With the high usage frequency of total parenteral nutrition solutions in hospital practice, many LVPs are now available containing high concentrations of dextrose. These and other highly viscous solutions are filtered through several filter assemblies since one assembly will not permit the passage of the entire contents of a viscous solution. However, the total volumes and number of containers per medium remain the same as required for non-viscous solutions. Half of the total number of membranes used are incubated in each medium.

Commentary: While the MF method offers distinct advantages over the DT method, the risk of extraneous contamination is greatly increased because of the manipulations additional to those employed in conducting the sterility test by direct transfer. Thus, extreme precautions must be followed in all the techniques involved in the MF method. Negative controls are especially recommended with the above methodology.

In transferring the container contents into the membrane filter funnel, great care must be used to avoid squirting solution directly onto the filter. Also, since this method is used to sterility test small-volume multidose parenterals containing antimicrobial preservatives, the membrane must be rinsed three times with USP Diluting Fluid A (100 ml) to ensure that the entire solute content has been washed through the membrane. The MF method is an excellent technique for the sterility testing of LVP solutions because low levels of contaminants in these dilute solutions are concentrated together upon the surface of one or two filters. If only the direct transfer method were available, even a representative sample of the LVP added to culture media would contain an insufficient number of microbial cells to harvest under the best of incubation conditions.

2. Membrane filtration of liquids immiscible with aqueous vehicles (less than 100 ml per container)

Summary of procedure: The required volume from 20 containers is transferred aseptically directly into one or two separate membrane filter funnels. After filtration via vacuum, the membrane is cut in half using aseptic procedure already described and incubated in 100 ml each of FTM and TSB. For immiscible liquids of high viscosity, aseptic addition of Diluting Fluid A is required to increase the flow rate. If the liquid has antimocrobial activity or contains an antimicrobial preservative, the filter is washed three times with 100 ml of the diluting fluid. Products containing lecithin, however, must use Diluting Fluid D containing the surface active agent Polysorbate 80 to enable the dispersion of the oily substance.

Commentary: Examples of products tested by this procedure are progesterone, testosterone propionate, and dromostanolone propionate in which the solvent is sesame oil or peanut oil.

3. Membrane filtration of ointments and oils soluble in isopropyl myristate

   Summary of procedure: Approximately 100 mg of sample from each of 20 containers is aseptically transferred to a flask containing 100 ml of sterile isopropyl myristate warmed to 44°C. The mixture is passed immediately through one or two membrane filter assemblies. After filtration, each membrane is washed with several 100—200 ml portions of Diluting Fluid D, then washed with 100 ml of Diluting Fluid A (see Table 1.4). The membranes are removed aseptically and immersed in FTM and TSB culture media containing Polysorbate 80. Test samples containing petrolatum are rinsed with Medium K (Table 1.5).

   Commentary: Isopropyl myristate was found to be a satisfactory solvent for dissolving petrolatum-based ointments without adversely affecting contaminants (23). Filter-sterilized isopropyl myristate is less toxic to microorganisms than heat-sterilized isopropyl myristate (24,25). Another solvent system that has been reported to aid in the sterility testing of parenteral fat emulsions is dimethyl-sulfoxide (DMSO) (26).

4. Membrane filtration of devices

   Summary of procedure: Diluting Fluid D is aseptically passed through each of 20 devices and at least 100 ml is collected from each device. The fluid is then filtered through a membrane filter, the membrane removed aseptically, cut in half, and each half placed in 100 ml FTM and 100 TSB, respectively.

Commentary: Several problems exist in the sterility testing of devices (27). Many devices are complex and cannot be manipulated easily. These would include prosthetic materials, large syringes, dispensing aids, and multiple-unit items. In such cases, direct transfer sterility testing may be the only practical method available. Devices must be handled in such a way so as to avoid accidental contamination. Correct aseptic technique becomes critical when sterility testing devices. The complexity of certain devices also affords greater probability of inadequate sterilization within tortuous or hard-to-reach sections of the device. Also, devices may be prepared in small lots of only a few units. Therefore, it is suggested that those concerned with the sterilization of devices periodically monitor their established sterilization cycles by means of long-term incubation of sterility test samples to assure the absence of viable microorganisms.

CONTROL IN STERILITY TESTING

Sterility testing provides an estimate of the probable extent of contamination of a lot of articles. Since it is only an estimate, it must be based on sound scientific principles. Such principles primarily involve the successful incorporation of controls within each and every test. Sterility testing is, however, only one component of control of sterility (sterility assurance in manufacture). In the broadest sense, control starts with the environmental, personnel, and sterilization conditions implemented during the manufacture of the sterile product. Control of the quality of the environment under which the sterility test is performed is of extreme importance. The training and experience of personnel conducting the sterility test must also be controlled with regard to their understanding, use, and attitude toward strict aseptic technique. These types of controls in manufacture will be discussed in a separate section. The types of control of sterility testing to be discussed in this section include the following: (a) positive control of the culture media, that is, the testing of the growth-promoting quality of each lot of media, (b) negative control of the culture media, that is, testing the sterility of the media, (c) control of the product itself, that is, obtaining knowledge about the bacteriostatic and/or fungistatic activity of the product prior to its being subjected to a sterility test, and (d) specific controls when using the MF technique.

Positive Controls

The absence of growth in sterility test samples at the completion of the test indicates that the product is sterile insofar as assumptions and limitations of the test are considered, i.e., it meets the requirements of the test. However, this conclusion can be made only with the assurance that growth would have occurred during the sterility test period had microorganisms actually been present. The USP growth promotion test is designed to serve as a positive control for each lot of sterility test media. Each lot is inoculated with 10 to 100 of the microorganisms listed in Table 1.7. Growth of these microorganisms must occur in the appropriate medium within seven days' incubation. The evidence of growth in duplicate test containers compared with the same lot of medium containing no microbial inoculum qualifies the test medium to be used for sterility test purposes. The USP allows for the growth promotion test to be the positive control run simultaneously with the actual sterility test with the understanding that the test becomes invalid if the medium does not support the growth of the inoculated microorganisms. However, if tested media are stored, additional tests are prescribed for particular storage conditions.

Negative Controls

Negative controls consist of containers of culture media without addition of product sample or microbial challenge. The purpose of negative control samples is to verify the sterility of the medium before, during, and after the incubation period of the sterility test. If microbial growth is detected with a negative control, either the medium was not sterilized properly, contamination was introduced accidently during the test procedure, or there exists an inefficiency in the container or packaging system. If such microbial growth in a negative control occurs, and in the absence of evidence from the environmental monitor, equipment, or personnel of accidental contamination, it becomes a clear indication for retesting the product.

Bacteriostatic and Fungistatic Testing

If a sterility test is negative (no growth), there must be the assurance that growth was not inhibited by the antimicrobial properties of the product itself. The USP provides a procedure for determining the level of bacteriostatic and fungistatic activity of a product or material prior to its being tested for sterility by the direct transfer test. Basically, the procedure calls for adding

TABLE 1.7 Test Microorganisms Required by the USP for Use in the Growth Promotion Test For Each Lot of Media Used in Sterility Testing[d]

Medium	Test microorganisms[b]	Incubation temperature (°C)	Condition
Fluid thioglycollate	Bacillus subtilis (ATCC No. 6633)[c]	30—35	Aerobic
	Candida Albicans (ATCC No. 10231)	30—35	Aerobic
	Bacteroides vulgatus (ATCC No. 8482)[d]	30—35	Aerobic
Alternative thioglycollate	Bacteroides vulgatus (ATCC No. 8482)[d]	30—35	Anaerobic
Soybean-casein digest	Bacillus subtilis (ATCC No. 6633)[c]	20—25	Aerobic
	Candida albicans (ATCC No. 10231)	20—25	Aerobic

[a]ATCC cultures represent reference species and their use for compendial test is predicated on their not being subjected to procedures that may alter their properties. Such procedures include indefinite numbers of sub-cultures with no standardization of conditions. For this reason, the USP has proposed that seed lot culture techniques may be used and that the viable microorganisms used be not more than five passages removed from the reference species.

[b]Available from the American Type Culture Collection, 12301 Parklawn Drive, Rockville, MD 20852.

[c]If a spore-forming organism is not desired, use Micrococcus luteus (ATCC No. 9341) at the incubation temperatures indicated in the table.

[d]If a spore-forming organism is desired, use Clostridium sporogenes (ATCC No. 11437) at the incubation temperature indicated in the table.

TABLE 1.8 Inactivation of Bacteriostatic/Fungistatic Agents in Sterile Products Tested by the Direct Transfer Sterility Test

Agent	Method of inactivation
Mercurials	
Phenylmercuric nitrate (1:50,000 conc.)	10 ml FTM
Merthiolate (1:10,000 conc.)	10 ml FTM or 12 % sodium thiosulfate
Phenol	Adsorb on 0.1% Darco or 0.03% ferric chloride or dilute 0.5% phenol in 50 ml culture medium
Benzalkonium chloride	Lecithin and polysorbate 80
Sulfonamides	P-aminobenzoic acid
Penicillin	Penicillinase
Cephalosporins	Cephalosporinase
Streptomycin	Cysteine HCl 2% in acid medium
Cresol	Dilute 0.35% in 60 ml culture medium
Chlorobutanol	Dilute 0.5% in 40 ml culture medium
Barbiturates	Dilute to 0.2% in culture medium with a pH of about 7.0
Aminoglycosides	Acetyl-coenzyme A[a]

[a]A. S. Breeze and A. M. Simpson, An improved method using acetyl-coenzyme A regeneration for the enzymatic inactivation of aminoglycosides prior to sterility testing, *J. Appl. Bacteriol. 53*, 277 (1982).

product to containers of culture media in volumes corresponding to those that would be used for testing the product containing 10 to 100 of the microorganisms listed in Table 1.7 and comparing with medium-inoculum controls without the product. If the material possesses bacteriostatic or fungistatic activity, then the product-media will show decreased or no microbial activity compared to control culture media. If this is the case, then procedures must take place for the proper inactivation of these bacteriostatic/fungistatic properties. Either a suitable sterile inactivating agent must be found or the material and medium must be adequately diluted to overcome the static effects. If at all possible, the membrane filtration test should be applied for those materials found to be bacteriostatic or fungistatic. Where membrane filtration is used, similar comparisons are made of incubated filters through which product and suitable diluting fluid have been passed, each containing the same added microorganisms.

Specific inactivating or diluting methods used for a few drugs or drug products known to be bacteriostatic or fungistatic are listed in Table 1.8.

Controls for Membrane Filtration Techniques

The MF test relies on the ability to produce sterile equipment and to have aseptic conditions under which to conduct the test. Three basic control procedures are recommended in separate experiments:

1. The membrane filters are challenged after their sterilization cycle for their ability to retain microorganisms.
2. The exposure times for agar setting plates used to monitor the environment are validated.
3. The cleaning procedures used to remove bacteriostatic and/ or bactericidal residues from equipment following the MF test must be validated. This is especially important for the equipment involved in the sterility testing of antibiotics.

LIMITATIONS OF THE USP/NF REFEREE STERILITY TEST

The USP referee sterility test suffers from at least three limitations: (a) the invariant uncertainty that the small sample used in the test reliably represents the whole lot, (b) the inability of the culture media and incubation conditions to promote the growth of any and all potential microbial contaminants, and (c) the unavoidable problem of occasional accidental contamination of the sterility test samples. Ernst et al. (28) believe that impeccable control of three phases of the sterilization and sterility testing of parenteral products will alleviate many of the problems of sterility testing: (a) knowledge and understanding of the sterilization process, (b) avoidance of unfavorable environmental conditions during manufacture and testing, and (c) education of personnel in the procedures of sterility testing.

The Problem of Sampling and Statistical Representation

The probability of accepting lots having a given percent contamination is related to the sterility test sample size rather than to batch size (29). For example, if a batch if 0.1% contaminated (one non-sterile unit in 1000 units) and 10 units are sampled for a sterility test, the probability of finding one of those 10 samples to be the one contaminated unit in 1000 is not significantly different if the batch size were 1000, 2000, or 5000. Increasing the sample size from 10 to 20 to 50 units per batch, however, affects the probability of accepting the batch as sterile to a more significant degree than does the increase in batch size, assuming that the increase in batch size does not increase the level of contamination. This phenomenon is depicted in Table 1.9. The probability rate does not change as the batch size is increased, but does change as the sample size is increased. Of course, a key factor is that the contamination rate remains at 0.1% as the batch size increases. This, in reality, may not be true, especially for aseptically filled products. Hence, if the contamination rate increases with batch size, the probability of acceptance rate decreases for the same sample size.

The relationship of probability of accepting lots of varying degrees of contamination to sample size is given in Table 1.10 (30). Three details may be learned assuming the data in Table 1.10 to be real: (a) as the sample size is increased, the probability of accepting the lot as sterile is decreased; (b) at low levels of contamination, e.g., 0.1%, the odds of ever finding that one con-

TABLE 1.9 Probability of Accepting a Batch as Sterile Assuming the Contamination Rate to be Constant at 0.1%

Sterility test sample size	Batch size		
	1000	2000	5000
10	0.99	0.99	0.99
20	0.98	0.98	0.98
50	0.95	0.95	0.95

TABLE 1.10 Relationship of Probabilities of Accepting Lots of Varying Assumed Degrees of Contamination to Sample Size

Number of samples tested (n)	Probability of accepting the lot ("true" percent contamination of lot)					
	0.1	1	5	10	15	20
10	0.99	0.91	0.60	0.35	0.20	0.11
20	0.98	0.82	0.36	0.12	0.04	0.01
30	0.95	0.61	0.08	0.01		
100	0.91	0.37	0.01			
300	0.74	0.05				
500	0.61	0.01				

taminated sample in 1000 units are so small that one must face the fact that lots are going to be passed as sterile but somewhere, at some time, some patient is going to receive that non-sterile sample (even at a contamination rate of 1% with 20 sterility test samples, it must be realized that such a lot will be passed as sterile 82% of the time); and (c) realistically, a batch must be grossly contaminated for the sterility test to detect it. This fact was concluded at a 1963 conference on sterility testing in London (31) in which experts in sterility testing recognized that the lowest contamination rates that can be detected with 95% confidence are 28% with a sample size of 10, 15% with a sample size of 20, and 7% with a sample size of 40 units.

A sample size of 20 units is shown in Table 1.11. As an example, if it is assumed that only one unit in a batch of 100,000 units is contaminated (0.001%), the probability that the one contaminated unit is among the 20 sterility test samples taken at random is 0.0002, or 2 times in one million sterility tests. Table 1.12 presents an elaborative example of why dependence on sampling and sterility testing is, in fact, a futile attempt to prove the sterility of a lot.

A mathematical equation for calculating the probability (P) of releasing lots at different levels of contamination was developed by Armitage (32):

$$P = e^{-mv}$$

TABLE 1.11 Probability of Finding at Least
One Non-Sterile Unit in a Sample Size of 20
Subjected to a Sterility Test

Assumed percent non-sterile units in the lot	Probability of finding at least one non-sterile unit
0.10	0.01980
0.05	0.00995
0.02	0.00399
0.01	0.00199
0.005	0.00100
0.002	0.00040
0.001	0.00020

where m is the number of microorganisms per ml and v is the volume in ml of the test sample. For example, if 10 microorganisms
are present per 100 ml and the test sample is 100 ml (20 containers × 5 ml per container), the probability of releasing the lot
of this contaminated product is 0.0000454. Like the presented
data in the preceding tables, this equation shows that relatively
small sample sizes and/or low contamination levels result in lots
being judged to meet the sterility test requirements when, in fact,
a finite number of articles in the lot are non-sterile. Thus, claims
for low probability levels of non-sterility cannot realistically be
proven by the random sampling procedure of the USP sterility test
and sterility assurance must be achieved by appropriate control
measures in manufacture (see the following section, "Support
Techniques and Procedures for Sterility Assurance"). In fact,
with low levels of non-sterile units in a lot, any reasonable sampling plan would not provide realistic results (see Table 1.12).
This does not even consider the finite probability of inadvertent
contamination entering the product during the sterility test
procedures.

Problem of Supporting the Growth of
Microbial Contaminants

No single medium will support the growth of all microbial forms,
i.e., bacteria, molds, fungi, and yeasts. FTM will not recover

TABLE 1.12 Futility of Depending on Sampling and Sterility Tests for Sterility Assurance of a Lot[a]

	Probability of finding all negatives in samples of different sizes for various levels of contamination		
n	p = 0.1	p = 0.01	p = 0.001
10	0.35	0.90	0.99
20	0.12	0.82	0.98
40	0.01	0.69	0.96
160		0.20	0.85
640			0.53

[a]If the proportion of contaminated units in the lot is p, then the proportion of non-contaminated units in that lot is $1 - p$. Let that be designated q. Then the probability of finding non-contamination (i.e., acceptance) of that lot with taking n samples for testing if $(q)^n$.

If, where there is contamination, an acceptable level of acceptance is 1 in 100 lots tested, the probability where 0.1% of the lot is contaminated is achieved with 40 samples, but with lower contamination levels many more samples would be required, e.g., where 0.01% contaminated about 450 samples, where 0.001% contaminated about 4,500 samples, and where 0.0001% contaminated about 45,000 samples. This illustrates the futility of attempting to determine sterility levels (where low) by sterility tests alone.

Take the following example: If sterility tests have been done, using one medium and 20 samples on each occasion, and only two inoculated tubes showed growth, the proportion contaminated may be 2/200. However, if on the occasions the positive result was obtained, the test were repeated with another 20 samples each time, with negative results, the proportion contaminated may be 2/240, i.e., 0.0083, and the proportion not contaminated 0.9917. If that lot were contaminated to the determined level, to reduce the probability of acceptance to 1 in 100 would require about 550 samples to be taken. Not only is such a number not feasible, the probability of adventitious contamination in sterility tests (ranging from 0.2% to 3% of tests, see the section "Problem of Accidental Contamination" in this chapter makes even that possibility likely to yield an unreliable result.

very low levels of some aerobic spore formers such as *Bacillus subtilis* (13). Friedl (33) reported that TSB gave more efficient recovery of small numbers of *B. subtilis* and *Clostridium sporogenes* spores than in FTM. TSB, being strictly an aerobic medium, will not support the growth of the genus *Clostridia*. On the other hand, while FTM effectively supports the growth of various strains of *Clostridia*, it has been reported that sodium thioglycollate is toxic to *Clostridia* and this antioxidant should be replaced by cysteine hydrochloride (34).

TSB is incubated at 20−25°C to permit the adequate growth of facultative organisms such as enterobacteria (*Escherichia coli, Salmonella, Shigella, Proteus, Serratia marcescens,* and *Flavobacterium*) and many yeasts. FTM is incubated at 30−35°C to detect mesophilic bacteria. These sterility media, therefore, are not incubated at temperatures conducive to the growth of psychophiles (predominantly pseudomads) and thermophiles (predominately bacilli). According to Bruch (36), TSB and FTM do not contain the necessary nutritional ingredients to support the growth of obligate halophiles, osmophiles, or autotrophs.

Problem of Accidental Contamination

Growth that occurs in sterility test media must be ascertained to have originated from the test sample and not from the culture media or from an external source during the execution of the test. Such a determination can be made only to a limited extent. The use of negative controls eliminates one source of contamination, that being a result of non-sterile culture media. Thus, a positive sterility test result is concluded to be true (the test sample is contaminated) unless it can be shown to be false (contamination was accidently introduced during the test procedure). The problem of false positives is widespread and cannot be completely eliminated.

The percentage of false positive sterility test is reported to range from 0.2% to 3% (1,2,36). In a poll conducted by the author of this book, of 10 pharmaceutical companies involved in sterile product sterility testing, the range of inadvertent contamination found during sterility testing was 0.1% to 5%. The most common types of microbial contaminants found in false positive sterility test samples are listed in Table 1.13.

False positive sterility tests result also from contaminants located in the environment (air and surfaces), on people conducting the test (hands, breath, hair, clothing, etc.), or on the equip-

TABLE 1.13 Most Common Types of Contaminants
in False Positive Sterility Tests

Staphylococcus epidermidis

Gram positive rods (Bacillus and Clostridium)

Propionibacterium acnes

ment used in conducting the test (non-sterile membrane filter assemblies, scissors, forceps, filters, etc.). Contamination being
accidently introduced by the environment can be reduced significantly by performing a monitored environmental sterility test
in a laminar air flow (LAF) workbench (see this chapter's section
"Laminar Air Flow"). For example, Parisi and Borick (37) found
that the percentage of false positives during sterility testing fell
from 1.61% when done in conventional sterile rooms to 0.63% when
done in a LAF workbench. These same authors also reported that
2361 colonies were recovered on 765 agar settling plates located in
the conventional sterile room, while only 75 colonies were recovered on 299 agar settling plates located on a LAF workbench.
Thus, while LAF workbenches do not completely eliminate the incidence of contamination, they do significantly reduce the potential
problem provided the results from the settling plates are used to
indicate corrective actions.

The single largest contributor of accidental contamination in
sterility test samples is the person or people performing the test.
Personnel-induced accidental contamination primarily results from
a lack of strict adherence to good aseptic technique. Good aseptic
technique involves many considerations including apparel, eye-
hand coordination, concentration, and the desire to be as careful
as possible.

Accidental or adventitious contamination is one of the greatest
problems interfering in the interpretation of sterility test results in
hospital pharmacies (38). Bernick et al. (39) suggested that contaminated intravenous admixtures are not contaminated during the
admixture process but rather are contaminated from microorganisms
introduced during the sterility testing procedure. Such admixture processing should be carried out in appropriate hospital pharmacy facilities and not in the patient care areas. Sterility testing
should be an essential component in the monitoring of intravenous
solutions and admixtures in hospital pharmacy practice (40–45).
Several methods have been suggested for evaluating sterility of

intravenous admixtures (46—50). However, the problem of adventitious contamination and the limitations resulting from this problem that affect the interpretation of the sterility test must be recognized. The National Coordinating Committee for Large Volume Parenterals (NCCLVP) strongly recommends that suitable education programs in hospitals and colleges be developed to educate and train personnel involved in the parparation and administration of sterile medication (43). NCCLVP also recommends developing procedures for in-use testing of large-volume parenterals suspected of contamination.

SUPPORT TECHNIQUES AND PROCEDURES FOR STERILITY ASSURANCE

Because sterilization assurance is based on a probability function, sterility can never be proven unless the entire contents of a lot are subjected to a sterility test. Even this is not theoretically possible because of the need to use at least two different media for the test. Additionally, as has already been discussed, the sterility test itself has certain limitations. Therefore, product sterility cannot be tested with absolute assurance that every container of sterile product is sterile. However, assurance of product sterility can be achieved with a high degree of probability by the employment of and adherence to various procedures of which sterility testing is only an adjunct. These include: (a) sterilizer and sterilization method validation using physical and biological indicators, (b) impeccable control of the environmental conditions under which the parenteral product is manufactured particularly where aseptic processing is performed, and (c) thorough training of personnel of the strict aseptic techniques required for performing the sterility test. Any sterility test should be done in an environment no less controlled than that used for aseptic processing. An important part of long-range sterility assurance is adequate documentation of the validation, monitoring, and batch manufacturing procedures used.

Sterilizer and Sterilization Method Validation

The assurance of parenteral product sterility primarily depends upon the process used to sterilize the product. The greater the control of the process the greater the assurance of sterility. Sterilization process control involved knowledge and management of *process* variables such as temperature, pressure, concentration, humidity, load configuration, and filter integrity, and of *product* variables such as solution composition and viscosity, packaging specifications, and microbial content.

Four basic methods are employed to sterilize parenteral products. They are:

1. Heat, both wet (steam) and dry heat
2. Gas, primarily ethylene oxide
3. Radiation, primarily cobalt 60 gamma irradiation
4. Filtration through bacterial retentive membrane filters

The mechanics and engineering of each of these processes must be understood and properly controlled for the process to provide additional assurance of product sterility. Simmons (51) has elaborated on the engineering aspects of validating steam, dry heat, and ethylene oxide sterilizers. Filter integrity testing has been adequately described by Reti and Leahy (52). Once the sterilizing system itself has been qualified (i.e., for capability to achieve sterilization), then the process of sterilization can be validated. Validation of the process involves both physical and biological methodology. Physical methods include temperature measurement, gas concentration or irradiation dose monitoring, and the use of mathematical expressions such as the F value equation (53). Biological methods involve the employment of biological indicators to evaluate the ability of the sterilization process to destroy or eliminate an inordinately high concentration of known resistant microorganisms under conditions identical to those found in the sterilization of the actual parenteral product. They also are used to monitor a validated sterilization cycle.

Biological Indicators

Greater confidence in sterility assurance has arisen because of the increased acceptance and employment of biological indicators (BIs) during the development of the sterilization cycle or system (54). If the sterilization process is shown with a high degree of probability to destroy, say 10^6 spores of known resistance to the process, then a batch of parenteral product exposed to that same process will result in a sterile product. This may be roughly confirmed by the sterility test. BIs are microorganisms, usually spore forms, known to be as resistant to destruction by a given sterilization process as any microbial form known to man. BIs are used to verify the effectiveness of a sterilization process because if the process can destroy the BI of known concentration, it is assumed that the process will also destroy all other microbial contaminants potentially present in the product. Of course, this assumption is controversial and many experts question how far one can really depend upon it.

Microorganisms recognized by the USP as biological indicators for the various sterilization processes are given in Table 1.14. However, one is not restricted from employing other types of microorganisms as BIs if they better serve the needs of the particular process. Several species of *Bacillus* spore are known to be more resistant than the strain of *Bacillus subtilis niger* (ATCC 9372), the USP biological indicator for monitoring ethylene oxide sterilization (55). *B. pumilus* (ATCC 27142) has demonstrated the same degree of resistance to ethylene oxide as *B. subtilis niger* (56). Vegetative cells, rather than bacterial spores, are employed in testing and validating filtration sterilization. *Pseudomonas diminuta* (ATCC 19146) a vegetative organism selected for its small size (approximately 0.3 µm), is the organism of choice for evaluating the retention ability of 0.2 µm sterilizing membrane filters.

The USP provides a general description of BIs. BIs are available either as liquid suspensions or as dried preparations on carriers such as paper strips, glass, or plastic beads. BIs used as a spore suspension should be added to representative units or to units similar to those of the lot to be sterilized. The BI must demonstrate a challenge of the sterilization process that exceeds the challenge of the natural bioburden. BIs must be properly standarized so that the BI units in the lot all exhibit the same degree of resistance to the sterilization process when used in the same manner even if varying at different times within the dating period of the BI. The BI inoculum must be prepared under the supervision of trained microbiologists in order to maintain and standarize BI cultures of known purity, identity, and resistance. Every commercially prepared BI product must be labeled according to the relevant USP general notices on labeling as well as with its spore content and performance characteristics such as decimal reduction time (D value) under given sterilization parameters, directions for use, and recommendations for disposal.

Several interesting review articles have been written on the principles and applications of biological indicators. Borick and Borick (13) were the first authors to write a lengthy discussion on the use of biological indicators versus the use of regular sterility test samples. Bruch (35) presented a strong case for using BIs as a means of evaluating the probability of sterility of products sterilized by methods other than saturated steam under pressure. The USP sterility test is capable of detecting only high levels of product contamination on a consistent basis. Myers and Chrai (57)

TABLE 1.14 Performance Characteristics of Biological Indicators on Paper Strips

Culture	Sterilization process	D value	Approx. spore content	Survival time (not less than)	Kill time (not more than)
Bacillus stearothermophilus spores (ATCC 7953 or 12980)	Saturated steam at 121 ± 0.5°C	1.3–1.9 min	10^6	3.9 min	19 min
Bacillus subtilis subsp. *niger* (ATCC 9372)	Ethylene oxide at 54 ± 2° and relative humidity 60 ± 10%: 600 ± 30 mg/liter	2.6–5.8 min	10^6	7.8 min	58 min
	Dry heat at 160 ± 5°C	1.3–1.9 min	10^6	3.9 min	19 min
Bacillus pumilus (ATCC 27142)	Ionizing radiation				
	Wet preps.	0.16–0.24 Mrad	10^6	0.6 Mrad	2 Mrad
	Dry preps.	0.12–0.18 Mrad	10^6	0.45 Mrad	1.5 Mrad
General requirement		D ± 20%	10^6	3 D	10 D

reviewed the biology of microbial resistance and application of bioindicators in designing and monitoring sterilization cycles.

Caputo and Mascoli (58) suggested a four-step process in the design of a BI system for validating the efficacy of a sterilization cycle. In the first step, the microorganism to be used as the BI is selected and propagation procedures are developed to ensure the consistent production of a homogeneous population of BI with the desired resistance to the sterilization process. Second, the D value (the time required to reduce the microbial population by 90% or through one log cycle) is determined for the selected BI. Factors that must be considered and that affect the D value of a particular BI are discussed by Pflug and Odlaug (59). The third step in the design of a BI system is the actual evaluation of the sterilization process in destroying the BI employing a full load of product. Process parameters (temperature, gas concentration, humidity, radiation dose) are established during this step. Finally, a determination is made either of the amount of (log cycle) reduction required for the desired degree of probability or of the level of microorganisms to be used as a BI to validate the sterilization process, qualify the sterilization vessel, and, subsequently, monitor the sterilization process (60).

Environmental Control

Whenever possible, sterility tests should be performed in a test area that conforms to Class 100 conditions as described by Federal Standard Number 209B (61). Class 100 conditions mean that no more than 100 particles per cubic foot of size 0.5 μm or greater, as measured by electronic particle counters, shall be found in the measured area. A comparison of the classes of air cleanliness is provided in Table 1.15. However, so far, these classes refer to levels of particulate matter, not viable microorganisms.

Great strides have been made in recent years to help ensure that Class 100 conditions are met and that adequate microbial monitoring is effected in a sterility testing facility. Probably the greatest advancement was the discovery by Whitfield (62) in 1961 of the concept of laminar air flow.

Laminar Air Flow

Phillips and Miller (63) have succinctly described the concept of laminar air flow (LAF). The employment of LAF cabinets, workbenches, and rooms in the proper execution of the sterility test and other aseptic operations is essential. The air emitted from

TABLE 1.15A Guidelines for Air Cleanliness Classes

Type of facility		Class 100	Class 10,000	Class 100,000
Laminar air flow	Vertical flow room, vertical flow curtain units, vertical flow bench	Entire work area meets requirements at normal working height locations	Entire area meets requirements	Entire area meets requirements
	Crossflow room, tunnel room, wall-to-floor room, crossflow bench	First work locations meet requirements	Entire work area meets requirements. If particle generation, work locations and personnel are reasonably controlled.	Entire area meets requirements
Non-laminar air flow	Conventional clean room	Will *not* meet requirements under operation conditions	Can be upgraded to meet requirements by placing laminar air-flow devices within the room and continuously filtering the recirculating air. Personnel and operation restrictions and janitorial maintenance are also required.	Will meet requirements with strict observation of rules governing personnel, operations, garmenting, and janitorial procedures.
	Computer rooms	Will meet requirements with personnel restriction and janitorial maintenance	Entire area meets requirements	Entire area meets requirements

Source: Courtesy of Liberty Industries, East Berlin, Connecticut.

TABLE 1.15B

Max. number of particles per cubic ft. 5.0 μm and larger	Class	Max. number of particles per cubic ft. 5.0 μm and larger
100	100	0
1,000	1,000	7
10,000	10,000	65
20,000	20,000	130
100,000	100,000	700
1,000,000	1,000,000	6,500

Source: Courtesy of Liberty Industries, East Berlin, Connecticut.

LAF equipment is claimed to be 99.97% free from microbial contamination. This level is based upon the removal of dioctylphthalate particles of size 0.3 μm and larger. Thus, although a theoretical 0.03% contamination level exists when using LAF equipment, the air within the confined area of the workbench or cabinet is considered to be sterile.

LAF equipment can deliver clean air in a vertical, horizontal, or curvilinear direction. The principles of vertical and horizontal airflow are shown in Figures 1.7 and 1.8, respectively. Room air is sucked into the equipment and passes through a prefilter which removes large-sized air contaminants. A blower then forces the prefiltered air through a second filter system in the LAF unit called a High Efficiency Particulate Air (HEPA) filter (Figure 1.9). Air passing through the HEPA filter not only is 99.97% particle free, but also moves with uniform velocity along parallel flow lines. Proper aseptic procedures to be practiced while working at the laminar flow workbench during sterility testing are listed in Appendix IV (64).

Quality control procedures must be adopted to evaluate and monitor the quality of the LAF hood environment. This includes monitoring with particles and microorganisms. Since LAF hoods are supposed to provide Class 100 air, they should be certified that this standard is met. Certification is done immediately after installation of new HEPA filters and at periodic intervals, usually

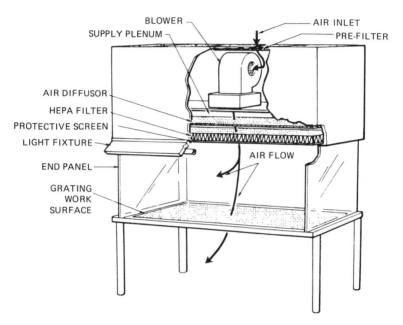

FIGURE 1.7 Vertical laminar air flow bench. (Courtesy of Liberty Industries, East Berlin, Connecticut.)

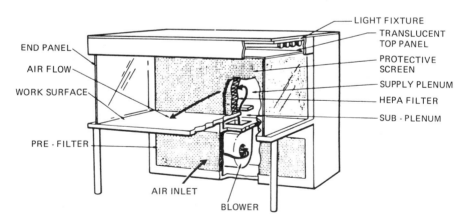

FIGURE 1.8 Horizontal laminar air flow bench. (Courtesy of Liberty Industries, East Berlin, Connecticut.)

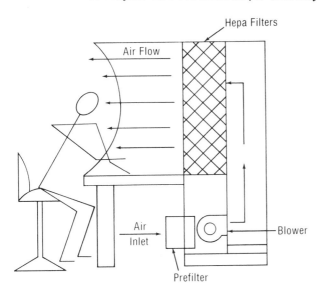

FIGURE 1.9 Direction of air flow in a laminar air flow work station. (Courtesy of Liberty Industries, East Berlin, Connecticut.)

every 6 to 12 months. The velocity of HEPA-filtered air is measured using an air velometer. Air velocity at all parts of the filter should be 90 ± 20 feet per minute. Air quality is evaluated using particle counters, microbial air samplers, and agar settling plates. The efficiency of the HEPA filter in removing particulate and microbial contamination is evaluated by employing the dioctylphthalate (DOP) test. This is a universally acceptable challenge test for HEPA filters. DOP is a volatile liquid, which, under pressure, converts to a vapor or smoke having a size range of 0.28 to 0.4 μm. The DOP smoke is introduced at the supply plenum. A photometer probe then scans the entire HEPA filter surface. Any leaks in the filter will permit the DOP smoke to escape and this will be detected by the photometer. Several references are available describing the testing of laminar flow equipment (65–67). Phillips and Runkle (68) have published a comprehensive review of the biomedical applications of laminar air flow.

For most sterility testing operations, horizontal laminar air flow units appear to be superior to vertical flow hoods because the air movement is less likely to wash organisms from the operators' hands or equipment into the sterility test media (63). However, the operator must be specifically trained on how to utilize the air flow properly. HEPA filtered air will not sterilize the surface of a contaminated object. It will only maintain sterility or cleanliness of an already sterile or clean object. All surfaces of the LAF hood except the HEPA filter itself must be thoroughly disinfected before placing any item inside the hood. All materials must be disinfected prior to introducing such materials onto the surface of the laminar air flow workbench. For example, all glassware, containers, and other articles whose surfaces are non-sterile must be wiped thoroughly with a disinfectant solution before placing these items in the LAF unit. Sterile materials enclosed in protective packaging, such as plastic bags contained in polyethylene outer pouches, disposable syringes, sterile scissors and forceps wrapped in aluminum foil, wrapped membrane filter units, etc., may be introduced into the LAF unit by removing the outer protective package at the edge of the workbench before placing the sterile item on the workbench surface. Understanding of the laminar air flow pattern is very important in order to avoid turbulence and blockage of HEPA filtered air reaching the critical work site.

Design and Maintenance of Aseptic Areas

The USP states that the principal sources of contamination are the air and water in the aseptic processing area and the personnel, materials, and equipment involved in the processing. Avis (69) has described what considerations must be met in the design, construction, and implementation of a sterile products facility. The design and operation of clean rooms have been the subjects of a major textbook (70). All areas must be designed and constructed to permit adequate cleaning, efficient operation, and comfort of personnel. Process flow must follow a plan in which product and personnel move to increasingly clean environments. An example of a process flow diagram is found in Figure 1.10 (69).

Ceilings, walls, and floors in the aseptic processing area must be sealed for ease and thoroughness in washing as well as treatment with disinfecting products. All counters, cabinets, and sinks should be constructed of stainless steel. All equipment, service lines and facilities, and other essential room fixtures should be constructed in such a manner to permit ease of cleaning and disinfecting and to prevent the accumulation of dust and dirt.

Several engineering features of a well-designed aseptic area are listed in the USP. However, newer proposals emphasize the principles involved rather than describe in detail the features of the

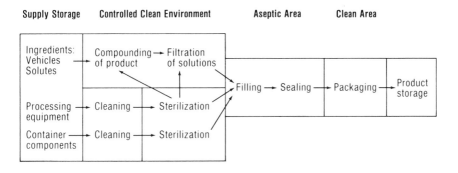

FIGURE 1.10 Diagram of flow of materials through a production department. (From Ref. 69.)

facility. The following considerations list a number of features, not all of which are necessarily applicable to any particular facility:

1. Hoods, cabinets, and other enclosures to serve as a primary barrier around the process, while the aseptic room itself serves as a secondary barrier
2. Maintenance of differential positive air pressures to prevent inward leakage of air
3. Effective filtration of air supplied to the primary and secondary barriers
4. Provision of air locks and/or air showers at the entrances to rooms, a gowning room, and adequate space for personnel garment storage
5. An effective intercommunication system and a suitable room arrangement to minimize traffic

An appropriate program should be established initially to qualify aseptic areas and equipment and routinely to monitor the integrity of the measures. The least controlled and potentially greatest source of contamination originates from the people working in the aseptic processing area and conducting the sterility test procedures. Training of personnel to minimize potential contamination arising from people is discussed in the following section, "Personnel Training."

Methods of Evaluating the Environment

A number of proven, quantitative viable and non-viable microbial counting methods are available for evaluating and monitoring the environment under which sterility tests are conducted. These methods can be further divided into air and surface sampling methods.

Air sampling methods

1. Slit-air sampler: This is a device that collects viable airborne microbial and particulate contamination (see Figure 1.11). A 150 mm sterile agar plate containing a layer of sterile agar, usually trypticase soy agar, is placed on a circular plate in the slit-air device and the cover containing the slit is secured above the agar plate. The speed of the plate rotation and the volume of air sampled can be adjusted to record the desired rate and degree of contamination of the air environment. The slit-air sampler is one of the most widely used monitoring methods for sterile manufacturing and quality control environments.

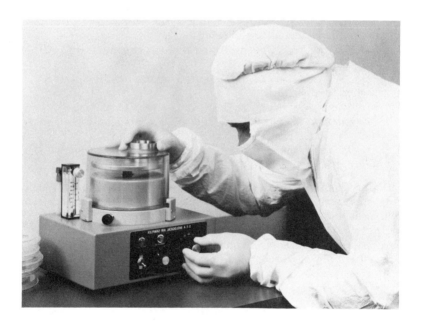

FIGURE 1.11 Slit-to-agar biological air sampler. (Courtesy of New Brunswick Scientific Co., Inc., Edison, New Jersey.)

2. Liquid impinger: This device works by using a vacuum source to such in air at a high velocity through an isotonic impingement fluid, then passing the fluid through a membrane filter by vacuum and incubating the filter on an agar plate. While liquid impingement thoroughly collects viable microbial contamination within a given cubic foot of air, it suffers two primary disadvantages. One disadvantage is the fact that microbial counts may be underestimated because the high velocity of impingement kills many organisms upon impact with the agar surface. The other disadvantage is the problem of air locks occurring at the filter surface as the impingement and diluting fluids are being vacuum filtered.

3. Electronic air particle counters: These instruments count all particles in the environment and cannot differentiate between viable and non-viable particles. These counters are especially useful in determining the number of particle

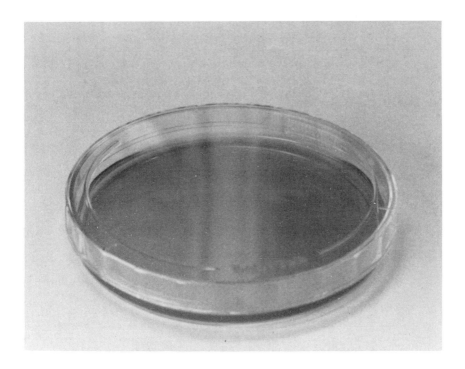

FIGURE 1.12 Agar settling plate.

counts per cubic foot to classify the cleanliness of a particular room or area.

4. Settling plates: These represent the simplest means of evaluating the microbiological quality of air. A 100 × 20 mm petri dish containing trypticase soy agar or other suitable medium is placed in a sampling location with the lid removed and placed as shown in Figure 1.12. The time period of sampling is controlled—it is usually 30 minutes—before the lid is placed over the medium and the plate incubated, usually at 32°C for 48 hours. Colonies are counted and many different locations within the sterility testing and manufacturing areas can be controlled and compared for microbial contamination. The major disadvantage of this method is that the volume of air sampled and represented on the agar plate is unknown.

5. Centrifugal air sampler: This device (see Figure 1.13) is the newest of the methods used to determine airborne contamination. Airborne microbes approximately 16 inches above the sterile drum housing are drawn toward the impeller blades. Then, owing to the applied centrifugal force, 4014–4178 rpm, the microbial particles are impacted at high velocity onto the agar surface of the agar strip wound around the impeller blades. After incubation the strips are counted and the results reported as colony-forming units per unit volume. The air capacity sampler per minute is 40 liters. In a comparative study of airborne microbial recovery rates (71), the RCS centrifugal air sampler was found to be significantly more efficient than the slit sampler and the liquid impinger. The centrifugal air sampler samples a greater area (1.2 cubic feet) versus 0.5 cubic feet sampled by the slit sampler (72).

Surface sampling methods

1. Rodac plates: These are specially built petri plates in which sterile culture media, usually trypticase soy agar containing Polysorbate 80 and lecithin, is poured onto a baseplate until a convex surface extends above the rim of the baseplate (see Figure 1.14). Once the molten agar has solidified, the agar surface can be gently pressed against a selected surface, e.g., the surface of a laminar airflow workbench. The lid is replaced and the plate incubated for the required length of time at a controlled temperature (commonly 48 hours at 32°C). Surface contamination can be quantified by counting the colonies after incubation. The presence of Polysor-

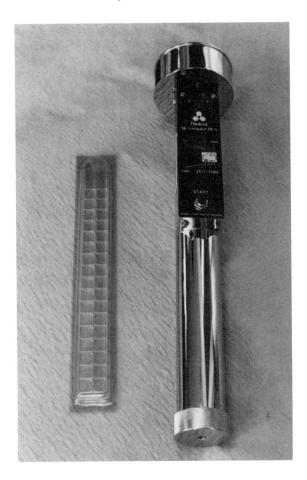

FIGURE 1.13 Biotest RCS centrifugal air sampler.

bate 80 and lecithin serves two purposes, one to aid in the complete contact and removal and microbes from the sampled surface and the other to permit cleaning of the sampled area with water and/or a disinfectant solution.

2. Swab-rinse test: This is a simple surface sample method employing sterile cotton swab tips to sample locations that are unwieldy for Rodac plates or difficult to reach. The swabs are then placed into tubes of culture media or, for microbial quantification, are mixed with sterile water and a sample of the water placed on a solid agar plate.

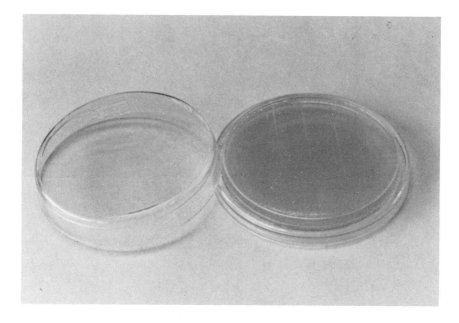

FIGURE 1.14 Convex surface of Radac agar plate.

Many of these environmental testing procedures and a suggested
program for determining microbiological burden and action levels
for both non-sterile and sterile environments can be found in a
paper by Dell (73). Tables 1.16 and 1.17 are reproduced from his
paper. These guidelines can be useful in establishing a program
design for environmental monitoring specific to the history, conditions, and needs of any particular manufacturing and sterility
testing facility.

The ultimate purpose of environmental control of microbial contamination is to minimize the potential for inadvertent product
contamination. The lesser the potential for contamination, the
greater the assurance that the product is sterile. The sterility
test then can be used primarily as a confirmation of the sterility
already built into the product.

Personnel Training

Most inadvertent contamination found in the sterility testing of
parenteral products originates from the personnel involved in the

TABLE 1.16 Example of an Environmental Testing Program for Monitoring a Sterile Production Facility

Element	Membrane filtration	Most probable number	Pour plate	Rodac	Swab	Settle plate	Slit air	Other[a]	Frequency[b]
Walls and floors									
Sterility test area				X	X				M
Controlled areas				X	X				M
Critical areas				X	X				M
HEPA-filter air									
Controlled areas						X	X	DOP	M
Critical areas						X	X	DOP	B
Sterility test area						X	X	DOP	B
Components	X	X	X					MLT	H,B
In-process bulk	X	X	X					MLT	H,B
Production equipment									
Tanks					X				
Hoses and lines	X							DM,VF	M
Filling equipment								VF	
Compressed air and gas	X							ORG	H
Potable water	X	X	X					LF	D
Deionized and distilled water	X	X	X					PT	D
HEPA filter						X	X	V,DOP	M
Finishing supplies	X		X						H

a*MLT = USP microbial-limits test; DM = direct-method sterility test; VF = vial-fill or media-fill test; ORG = organic material (oil); LF = lactose fermentation (standard methods of analysis); PT = pyrogen test; V = velometer; DOP = dioctylphthalate smoke test.
b M = monthly; B = batch or shift; H = history; D = daily.
Source: From Ref. 73.

TABLE 1.17 Example of Guidelines (Action Levels) for Environmental Monitoring of Sterile Production Elements

Sterile-processing location[a]	Bacteria (per sq cm)			Mold (per sq cm)		
	SP	SA	SP	SA	SP	SA
Controlled areas (Class 10,000–100,000)						
Walls, floors, equipment; swab or Rodac		<1				<1
Assembly rooms		<10				<2
Critical areas (Class 100)						
Walls, floors, equipment; swab or Rodac		0				0
Controlled areas—air sampling[b]						
Component preparation areas	10	100	2			25
Transfer areas	2	25	1			10
Gowning rooms	2	25	1			10
Wash booths	5	50	2			10
Staging areas	50	500	10			100
Compounding rooms	2	25	1			10
Critical areas—air sampling[b]						
Filling rooms	2	10	0			2
Sterility test laboratory	1	<1	0			0
Water[c]		<1/ml	0/ml			

[a]Controlled areas: sampled following sanitizing and prior to use.

[b]Air sampling: settling plate-exposed for 30 min or slit-to-agar sampling at a rate of 28.3 liters air/min for 30 min.

[c]Water tests same as for non-sterile manufacturing. Microbial count refers to "at time use."

Source: From Ref. 73.

testing program. Nearly all personnel-induced accidental contamination is produced either by the ignorance of an individual
who has not been adequately trained in good aseptic technique or
by the carelessness of an individual who has been trained in good
aseptic technique. Thus, learning and applying aseptic technique
not only requires physical and intellectual abilities, but also involves the development and persistence of a correct mental attitude. The latter is very difficult to instill. No one in a free society can be forced to comply to rigid standards. Supervisors
who hire personnel to perform sterility tests should abide by three
general rules:

1. The supervisor himself must recognize the need to comply
   with strict aseptic technique.
2. The supervisor should hire people who are willing to be
   trained and to accept and follow aseptic procedures.
3. The supervisor must effectively communicate and exemplify
   the importance of adhering to aseptic technique, without
   breeding ill feelings and subsequent poor attitudes.

Current good manufacturing procedures (CGMPs) (Section
211.25) contain several statements regarding the training of
people engaged in the manufacture, processing, packaging, and
holding of drug products. Personnel will be trained not only to
perform sterility tests, but also to understand CGMPs and standard operating procedures as they relate to sterility testing.
 Training in correct aseptic technique includes five general areas
of education:

1. General rules to follow when a person is working in a clean
   or sterile room
2. Proper gowning technique
3. Proper use of the laminar air flow workbench or other
   clean environment
4. Specific operations and manipulations while actually performing the sterility test, which are essential in maintaining
   asepsis
5. Proper clean-up at the conclusion of the test

No matter how well constructed a sterile or clean room may be, it
cannot compensate for people working in the area who are untrained with respect to sources of contamination. DeVecchi (74)
has published 29 rules or restrictions to be aware of when training
people to work in sterile environments. These are listed in Table
1.18.

TABLE 1.18 General Rules and Procedures for Working in a
Sterile Environment

---

1. Before entering any sterile environment, personnel should
    understand the responsibilities of their position and know
    clean-room techniques and system operations.

2. Personnel must react effectively in emergencies such as:
    fire outside or inside the sterile room, explosions outside or
    inside the sterile room, electrical failure, breaking of con-
    tainers holding toxic or non-toxic substances, illness or
    injury.

3. Everyone who enters the sterile area must be familiar with
    with gowning technique.

4. Without exception, all personnel working, supervising, con-
    trolling, or maintaining a sterile room should wear the
    approved sterile-room garments.

5. No sterile-room garment may be used a second time without
    being rewashed and resterilized.

6. Everyone working in sterile areas must know the disinfection
    and sterilization procedures.

7. Once inside a sterile room, personnel should avoid returning
    to the air lock. If a worker must go to the restroom, com-
    plete resterilizing and regarmenting are necessary prior to
    re-entering the clean room.

8. Plastic bags for disposal of used garments should be pro-
    vided in the air locks adjacent to powdered-antibiotic filling
    or preparation areas. The garments may be transported in
    these bags to the laundry area without risk of cross-contam-
    ination between product and personnel.

9. For reasons of comfort and efficiency, establish a minimum
    number of people to be allowed in the air locks at any one
    time.

10. No personnel articles (purses, bags, etc.) are permitted
    inside the sterile rooms or air locks.

11. No one who is physically ill, especially with a stomach or
    respiratory disorder, may enter sterile rooms or sterile areas.

12. All verbal communication with people outside of the sterile
    room should be accomplished through use of the intercom—
    never through air locks or passthroughs.

TABLE 1.18 (Continued)

13. The sterile-room doors must be kept closed at all times. They may open only to admit one person or product at a time.

14. Smoking is prohibited inside sterile rooms and neighboring rooms.

15. The use of cosmetics, wigs, makeup, long nails, rings, watches, etc., is prohibited in sterile rooms.

16. All materials, containers, or equipment introduced into the sterile room must be subjected to stringent sterilization procedures prior to entering the sterile areas.

17. Only long-fibered materials may be used for cleaning in sterile areas. Synthetic materials are suggested. Mops, brooms, and other customary cleaning equipment should not be used in sterile areas.

18. Paper in any form (except paper produced expressly for sterile-room standards, and meeting Class 100 conditions as delineated in Federal Standard 209B) is not allowed in sterile rooms.

19. Under no circumstances should food or beverages be introduced into a sterile room.

20. No pencils or ball-point pens should be used in a sterile room. Magic markers or felt-tip pens are suggested.

21. When it is necessary that paper forms be used in sterile areas, the form should be shielded with a clean plastic covering that has a window exposing the area on which the operator is writing.

22. Two different products are not to be processed in the same sterile room at the same time.

23. Antibiotic products in a powder form or liquid products of any kind should be manufactured in areas designated specifically for that purpose.

24. Disinfection and cleaning of the room must be completed at scheduled times. All personnel in the sterile room should know the cleaning and disinfection techniques used.

25. The sterile room must be kept clean at all times. Personnel, equipment, and materials introduced into a sterile room should be kept to a minimum.

TABLE 1.18 (Continued)

---

26. Once production runs are discontinued, any material from the previous production run should be removed from the sterile room to avoid cross-contamination.

27. Cleaning and/or disposal of all support material should be done after each workday.

28. Sterile-room furniture should be of simple design. No chair covers or chairs with foam parts are allowed in sterile areas. Tables should be stainless steel and without drawers. Equipment should be properly covered. No equipment with belt-driven or high-speed moving parts should be permitted in a sterile environment unless that equipment has proper covering.

29. All materials, containers, equipment, etc., authorized for sterile-room use must be labeled so as to be easily identified by clean-room personnel.

Source: From Ref. 74.

The importance of gowning may be emphasized best by reference to a statement by Abdou (75):

A room in which people work cannot be made sterile, regardless of how closely instructions concerning personal hygiene are followed. Twenty percent of the cutaneous flora is located so deep within the follicular channels that it cannot be reached by normal disinfection procedures. Such a reservoir or organisms ensures that the surface flora will quickly reestablish itself after the usual treatment of the skin with disinfectants. The epidermal fragments that people shed carry microorganisms, and the more vigorous the physical activity, the more the shedding. The skin of a healthy adult can shed betwee two and six million colony-forming units in one-half hour of vigorous activity.

Thus, the use of particulate-free gowning materials and adherence to strict gowning procedures will help to assure that the human body and clothing will not be a source of contamination. However, Brier et al. (76) reported that employment of clean room gowning did not affect the contamination rate of admixtures compounded in a hospital pharmacy. What was important was that I.V. admixtures were compounded using a laminar air flow workbench.

Proper use of the LAF working environment in the content of this discussion refers to the movement and manipulations of hands and objects in the hood without interfering or interrupting the flow of sterile air onto articles which must be kept sterile. Procedure 8 in Appendix IV should be reiterated at this point before reading further. Opening containers, devices, or other articles in which a sterile surface or pathway will be exposed should be completed so that the sterile part faces the HEPA filtered air. Moving, tilting, or otherwise manipulating open containers must be accomplished without fingers and hands either making contact with the exposed opening or coming between the opening and the airstream pathway. Using sterility test aids such as sterile forceps, scissors, filters, and other devices must be handled with care so as not to touch-contaminate the article. Whenever the operator suspects that he has accidentally touched a sterile surface, that article should be discarded. Fingers that have been disinfected and, subsequently, make contact with a nonsterile object should be disinfected again with a suitable disinfectant solution or foam. The most important aspect of working in an LAF workbench is mental concentration on the task at hand, always realizing where the hands are in relation to the HEPA filtered airstream and the critical work sites.

Operator training on the actual sterility testing procedures means the learning of the standard operating procedure (SOP) written for the sterility test to be executed. This step is probably the most time-consuming component of the training process. The operator will work closely with an experienced supervisor or other trainer for the length of time required for the operator to learn the SOP and perform the test without error in procedure and/or technique. The rate of false positive sterility test samples will be ascertained for each new operator and, obviously, a certain acceptable rate must be attained for the operator to be entrusted with future sterility test responsibility. Each sterility testing facility should set up a monitoring program to check periodically the rate of false positive samples produced by each operator. Hospital pharmacies that prepare intravenous admixtures and other sterile products should also maintain training programs for their sterile products technicians. Organized training programs based on national standards are being considered by the American Society of Hospital Pharmacists (77).

Regardless of how well a person is trained in the procedural aspects of conducting sterility tests, that individual must also possess the right mental attitude toward the responsibility and implications at hand. Otherwise, a mediocre or poor attitude will result in carelessness, indifference, and, ultimately, errors in technique. A right attitude must be present in the individual at the beginning, and then maintained and motivated through supervisory encouragement and reward.

ALTERNATIVES TO THE COMPENDIAL STERILITY TEST

The limitations of the USP/NF sterility test have already been addressed. They include the large sampling error due to the very small sample size tested for sterility, the problem of inadvertent contamination during sterility testing, and the difficulty in recovering low-level contamination and contribute to reasons for finding alternative procedures to the USP test as it is described for a reference test. Another reason for searching for alternative sterility test procedures is to fill the need of hospital pharmacies and other laboratory environments in which sterile solutions are prepared or manipulated in some manner. The USP referee sterility test is too time-consuming and costly to be used routinely in hospital practice, especially with the enormous numbers of intravenous admixture solutions being prepared.

At least two basic methods have been used for sterility testing in hospital practice. One involves the sampling of an aliquot volume of solution from an I.V. bottle (39), while the other method involves the filtration of all of the remaining portion of the bottle's contents through a closed filter system (78). In the first method, an aliquot sample is added to a concentrated broth solution such as double-strength brain-heart medium, FTM, or other suitable culture medium, or, if it is feasible, the concentrate is added in a volume equal to the contents of the bottle, as it is. The container is incubated, then inspected for the presence of microbial growth. The advantage of this method is its simplicity and cost. Its disadvantages include its potential for accidental contamination and the inability of one culture medium to promote the growth of all potential microbial contaminant, especially in large-volume solutions because of the high dilution factor. In the second method, a special device [Steritest, Millipore (Figure 1.15), or IVEX-Abbott (Figure 1.16)] is designed to permit in a closed system the filtration of the entire contents of a bottle through a plastic presterilized unit containing a $0.22-0.45$ μm membrane filter. Trypticase soy broth is then added aseptically and the unit is incubated intact. This closed system was designed to reduce the rate of false positives and to provide a more convenient method of sterility testing large-volume solutions and admixtures in hospitals (79).

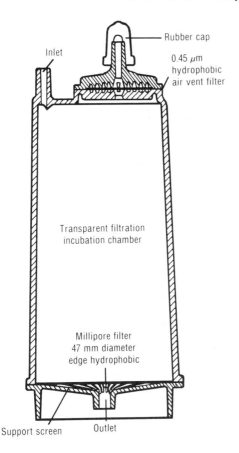

FIGURE 1.15 Steritest chamber (Millipore Corp., Bedford, Massachusetts, From Ref. 78.)

Disadvantages of the filter device system are its relatively high cost and some concern about its sensitivity to low level contamination.

Posey et al. (80) compared these two methods for detecting microbial contamination in 1 liter plastic bags of parenteral nutrition solutions containing between 1 and 1000 bacterial or yeast organisms per ml. Ten ml aliquots from each bag were withdrawn and injected into blood culture bottles. The remaining fluid was filtered through the Addi-chek system. The aliquot sampling method

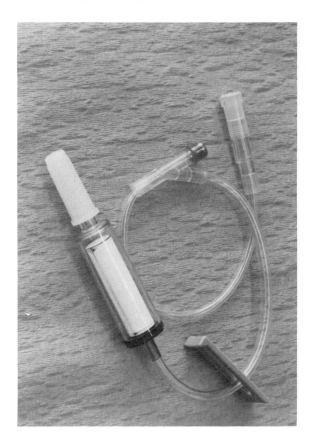

FIGURE 1.16 IVEX-2 device. (Courtesy of Abbott Laboratories, North Chicago, Illinois.)

consistently detected each of the organisms tested at levels of 100 organisms per liter and above. The filtration method consistently detected all levels of contamination. The authors concluded that the aliquot sampling method was inexpensive and easy to use, but failed to detect some contaminated solutions. The filtration method detected all levels of contamination, but is more costly in both time and money, and its reliability needs additional assessment.

The Addi-chek system was compared in a like manner with the IVEX-2 Filterset in the sterility testing of intravenous admixtures (81). Both filter systems were comparable in detecting low level microbial contamination, but the IVEX-2 system can be used to test for contamination when used as an in-line filter for patient administration of I.V. fluids. Like the aliquot sampling method, the IVEX-2 system is less expensive than the Addi-chek system. Both IVEX-2 and the method of combining equal volumes of product sample and double-strength trypticase soy broth were found to be more reliable and sensitive than Addi-chek in detecting low-level bacterial contamination in I.V. solutions, especially Dextrose 5% (82,83). Addi-chek sterility testing consumed more time in processing, allowing Dextrose 5% time to exert an inhibitory effect on microbial growth. Also, Addi-chek uses a 0.45 μm membrane filter while IVEX-2 contains a 0.22 μm filter.

A modification of the Addi-chek device to be used as an alternative to the membrane filtration method for the sterility testing of antibiotics has been described (84). The modified unit is shown in Figure 1.17. Two separate spikes are connected to a two-way valve that prevents the siphoning of the antibiotic into the rinse and media line. The rinse and media line is used to transfer the rinse solution to the canister. The rinse removes inhibitory residual antibiotic from the canister so that the contaminating microbes that may have been deposited on the filter may grow. After the rinse procedure, one canister is filled with TSB and the other with FTM. This system has been found to recover organisms with equal efficiency (as compared with the USP membrane filtration method) and, since it uses a closed, presterilized, and ready-to-use system, greatly reduces the chances of operator error and accidental contamination.

The use of an in-line 0.22 μm membrane filter set to test the sterility of I. V. solutions and administration sets (under actual use conditions) was found to have valuable application in I. V. fluid administration (85). Following filtration, brain-heart infusion broth was introduced into the filter chamber and the filter sets were incubated. Microbial contamination was found for all contaminated I. V. solutions and administration sets. No false positive results were found.

Sterility testing of small-volume unit dose parenteral products in the hospital environment was suggested by Rupp et al. (86) using a sterile filter unit like those already described. Ten percent of each lot of unit dose syringes were filtered before adding FTM to the filter unit. The units were incubated and inspected for turbidity or color change.

A new and potentially practical hospital sterility test method for monitoring I. V. admixtures combines the membrane filtration technique and fluorescent microscopy (87). Solutions are filtered

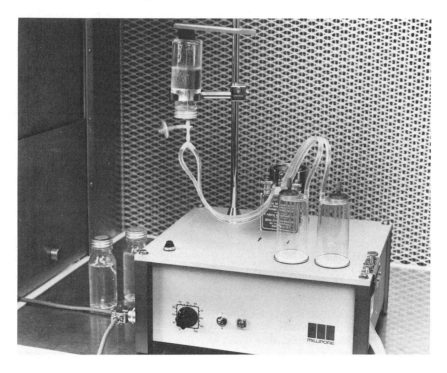

FIGURE 1.17 Diagram of modified Steritest unit. (From Reference 84.)

under vacuum through a 0.6 μm membrane filter. Then a staining compound (acridine orange solution) is poured onto the membrane and allowed to stand for three minutes. The stain is removed by vacuum and the membrane removed and mounted on a microscope slide. The membrane is examined within an hour with a light microscope fitted with an epifluorescent illuminator system. Any bacteria entrapped on the membrane surface will react with the fluorescent stain and, when illuminated with incident light, the total number of cells can be counted. The correlation between fluorescent counts and plate colony counts is excellent although the counts determined by fluorescence microscopy took only an hour or less while plate counting requires a 48-hour incubation. Sensitivity of this new method can be increased to levels as low as 25 organisms per ml and the technique can be automated.

Several alternative methods of sterility testing have been suggested in which neither aliquot sampling nor filtration is employed. One method suggested the addition of dehydrated broth powder (thioglycollate medium) to a random selection of bottles from each batch of infusion fluids before sterilization by autoclaving followed by incubation and daily inspection for turbidity (88). Another method employed the use of an electronic particle counter to detect contaminated culture media within 24 hours after adding contaminated membrane filters to the media (89). A recently propposed method for alternative sterility testing involved the use of luciferase assay for adenosine triphosphate (ATP) since detection of ATP indicates the presence of living cells (90). Each of these proposed sterility test alternatives offered one or more distinct advantages over the USP/NF sterility test either in terms of convenience, reducing the incidence of inadvertent contamination, or in significantly reducing the time required for detection of contaminated products. However, they are not necessarily alternatives to be preferred to a referee test in an advisory situation. Only in certain situations might one of these methods be a preferable alternative to the USP sterility test, especially in hospitals. For example, the luciferase ATP assay presents a very rapid method that can be used in septicemia investigations in which a large number of intravenous fluids must be tested as quickly as possible.

Several manufacturers expressed the desire to employ an automated sterility testing system. One system commercially available is the Bactec system (Johnston Laboratories). Its principle of operation is based on the detection of radioactive gas produced by decomposition of labeled substrates by microbial action. Samples of pharmaceutical product are withdrawn, inoculated into Bactec culture vials containing ^{14}C substrates, and incubated for 2–5 days. The Bactec instrument automatically tests the vials by analyzing the atmosphere in the vials. If the vial contains microorganisms, they will metabolize the ^{14}C substrates to product $^{14}CO_2$. A positive result will be indicated once a threshold level of $^{14}CO_2$ is exceeded. Models are available to test 60 culture vials per hour. The system offers expediency and convenience not characteristic of official sterility testing methods.

REFERENCES

1. C. C. Mascoli, Should end product sterility testing continue?, *Med. Device Diag.*, *3*, 8–9 (1981).

2. F. W. Bowman, The sterility testing of pharmaceuticals, *J. Pharm. Sci.*, *58*, 1301–1308 (1969).

3. P. M. Borick and J. A. Borick, Sterility of pharmaceuticals, cosmetics, and medical devices, *Quality Control in the Pharmaceutical Industry*, Volume 1 (M. S. Cooper, Ed.), Academic Press, New York, 1972, pp. 1–38.

4. A. Beloian, Methods of testing for sterility and efficacy of sterilizers, sporicides and sterilizing processes, *Disinfection, Sterilization, and Preservation*, 2nd Edition (S. S. Block, Ed.), Lea and Febiger, Philadelphia, 1977, pp. 11–48.

5. A. S. Outschoorn, USP standards for sterilization and sterility testing, *Developments in Industrial Microbiology*, Volume 18, Impressions, Inc., Gaithersburg, Maryland, 1977, pp. 387–397.

6. T. J. Macek, Proc. Ann. Mtg., Parenteral Drug Association, New York, 1970.

7. Code of Federal Regulations, Title 21, Section 610.12 for biologics and Section 436.20 for antibiotics, Superintendent of Documents, U.S. Government Printing Office, Washington, D. C.

8. L. K. Randolph and J. L. Climinera, Statistics, *Remington's Pharmaceutical Sciences*, 16th Edition, Mack Publishing, Easton, Pennsylvania, 1980, p. 126.

9. Military Standard Sampling Procedure and Tables for Inspection by Variables for Per Cent Deviation (MIL-STD-414), Superintendent of Documents, U.S. Government Printing Office, Washington, D. C., 1963.

10. S. Lin and L. Lachman, Quality assurance: process and dosage form control, *The Theory and Practice of Industrial Pharmacy*, 1st Edition, (L. Lachman, H. A. Lieberman, and J. L. Kanig, Eds.), Lea and Febiger, Philadelphia, 1970, p. 734.

11. C. B. Sampson, Quality control of the manufacturing process, *Statistics in the Pharmaceutical Industry* (C. R. Buncher and J. Y. Tsay, Eds.), Marcel Dekker, New York, 1981, p. 335.

12. J. Brewer, A clear liquid medium for the "aerobic" cultivation of anaerobics, *J. Bacteriol, 39,* 10 (1940).

13. J. E. Doyle, W. H. Mehrhof, and R. R. Ernst, Limitations of thioglycollate broth as a sterility test medium for materials exposed to gaseous ethylene oxide, *Appl. Micro., 16,* 1742–1744 (1968).

14. F. W. Bowman, M. White, and M. P. Calhoun, Collaborative study of aerobic media for sterility testing by membrane filtration, *J. Pharm. Sci.*, *60*, 1087–1088 (1971).

15. M. A. Abdou, Comparative study of seven media for sterility testing, *J. Pharm. Sci.*, *63*, 23–26 (1974).

16. F. W. Bowman, Application of membrane filtration to anti-biotic quality control sterility testing, *J. Pharm. Sci.*, *55*, 818–821 (1966).

17. A. G. Mathews, Optimal incubation conditions for sterility tests, *Dev. Biol. Stand.*, *23*, 94–102 (1974).

18. M. Pittman and J. C. Feeley, Proc. 7th International Congress Microbiol. Standardization, 7th Edition, E and S Livingstone, Edinburgh and London, 1962.

19. R. L. DeChant, D. Furtado, F. M. Smith, H. N. Godwin, and D. E. Domann, Determining a time frame for sterility testing of intravenous admixtures, *Amer. J. Hosp. Pharm.*, *39*, 1305–1308 (1982).

20. M. P. Calhoun, M. White, and F. W. Bowman, Sterility testing of insulin by membrane filtration: a collaborative study, *J. Pharm. Sci.*, *59*, 1022–1024 (1970).

21. G. W. Riedel and E. C. D. Todd, Sterility testing of large-volume aqueous pharmaceutical products (intraven-ous solution) by the membrane filtration technique, *Can. J. Pharm. Sci.*, *8*, 23–25 (1973).

22. D. A. Quagliaro, G. T. Spite, D. E. Guilfoyle, and W. E. Mestrandre, Development of culture vessel for sterility testing of other medical devices, *J. Assoc. Off. Anal. Chem.*, *62*, 695–699 (1979).

23. W. T. Sokolski and C. G. Chidester, Improved viable counting method for petrolatum-based ointments, *J. Pharm. Sci.*, *53*, 103–107 (1964).

24. K. Tsuji, E. M. Stapert, J. H. Robertson, and P. M. Waiyaki, Sterility test method for petrolatum-based ophthal-mic ointments, *Appl. Microbiol.*, *20*, 798–801 (1970).

25. K. Tsuji and J. H. Robertson, Microbial toxicity of isopropyl myristate used for sterility testing of petrolatum-based ophthalmic ointments, *Appl. Microbiol.*, *25*, 139–145 (1973).

26. A. M. Placenci, G. S. Oxborrow, and J. W. Davidson, Sterility testing of fat emulsions using membrane filtration and dimethyl-sulfoxide, *J. Pharm. Sci.*, *71*, 704 (1982).

27. J. H. Brewer and R. F. Schmitt, Special problems in the sterility testing of disposable medical devices, *Bull. Parenter. Drug. Assoc.*, *21*, 136–141 (1967).

28. R. R. Ernst, K. L. West, and J. E. Doyle, Problem areas in sterility testing, *Bull. Parenter. Drug. Assoc.*, *23*, 29–39 (1969).
29. L. F. Knudsen, Sample size of parenteral solutions for sterility testing, *J. Amer. Pharm. Assoc.*, *Sci. ed.*, *38*, 332–337 (1949).
30. J. H. Brewer, *Antiseptics, Disinfectants, Fungicides, and Sterilization*, 2nd Edition (G. L. Reddish, Ed.), Lea and Febiger, Philadelphia, 1957, pp. 160–161.
31. Proc. Round Table Conf. Sterility Testing, London, 1963, p. B31.
32. P. Armitage, A note on the safety testing of vaccines, *J. Hyg.* (Lond.), *69*, 95–97 (1971).
33. J. L. Friedl, Report on sporicidal tests, *J. Assoc. Off. Agric. Chem.*, *38*, 280–287 (1955).
34. D. A. A. Mossel and H. Beerens, Studies on the inhibitory properties of sodium thioglycollate on the germination of wet spores of *Clostridia*, *J. Hyg.*, *66*, 269–272 (1968).
35. C. W. Bruch, Levels of sterility: probabilities of survivors vs. biological indicators, *Bull. Parenter. Drug. Assoc.*, *28*, 105–121 (1974).
36. I. Scheibel and M. W. Bentzon, In Proc. III Int. Meeting of Biological Standardization, Opatija, Biostandards, Geneva, 1957.
37. A. N. Parisi and P. M. Borick, Proc. 7th Ann. Mtg. Assoc., *Contam. Contr.*, *7*, 24–26 (1968).
38. National Coordinating Committee on Large-Volume Parenterals: Recommended procedures for in-use testing of large-volume parenterals suspected of contamination or of producing a reaction in a patient, *Amer. J. Hosp. Pharm.*, *35*, 687–682 (1978).
39. J. J. Bernick, D. G. Brown, and J. E. Bell, Adventitious contamination of intravenous admixtures during sterility testing, *Amer. J. Hosp. Pharm.*, *36*, 1493–1496 (1979).
40. A. J. Hanson, R. M. Nighswander, and J. H. Verhulst, Monitoring of intravenous solutions, *Hosp. Formul.*, *8*, 17–21 (1973).
41. J. Whitbourne and K. West, Sterility Testing: how appropriate for the hospital?, *Med. Instru.*, *10*, 291–292 (1976).
42. W. A. Zellmer, Quality control in admixture services editorial, *Amer. J. Hosp. Pharm.*, *35*, 527–528 (1978).
43. Recommendations to pharmacists for solving problems with large-volume parenterals—1979, *Amer. J. Hosp. Pharm.*, *37*, 663–667 (1980).

44. M. H. Stolar, Assuring the quality of intravenous admixture programs, *Amer. J. Hosp. Pharm.*, *36*, 605 (1979).
45. National Coordinating Committee on Large-Volume Parenterals, Recommended guidelines for quality assurance in hospital centralized intravenous admixture services, *Amer. J. Hosp. Pharm.*, *35*, 678 (1978) and *37*, 645 (1980).
46. A. L. Hanson and R. M. Shelley, Monitoring contamination of in-use intravenous solutions using "total sample" techniques, *Amer. J. Hosp. Pharm.*, *31*, 733—735 (1974).
47. J. A. Buth, R. W. Coberly, and F. M. Eckel, A practical method of sterility monitoring of I. V. admixtures and a method of implementing a routine sterility monitoring program, *Drug. Intell. Clin. Pharm.*, *7*, 276—279 (1973).
48. R. B. Kundsin, C. W. Walter, and J. A. Scott, In-use testing of sterility of intravenous solutions in plastic containers, *Surgery*, *73*, 778—781 (1973).
49. R. Ravin, J. Bahr, F. Luscomb et al., Program for bacterial surveillance of of intravenous admixtures, *Amer. J. Hosp. Pharm.*, *31*, 340—347 (1974).
50. L. H. Sanders, S. A. Mabadeje, K. E. Avis et al., Evaluation of compounding accuracy and aseptic techniques for intravenous admixtures, *Amer. J. Hosp. Pharm.*, *35*, 531—536 (1978).
51. P. L. Simmons, The secret of successful sterilizer validations (Parts 13), *Pharm. Eng.*, *1* (Nov. 1980—July 1981).
52. A. R. Reti and T. J. Leahy, Validation of bacterially retentive filters by bacterial passage testing, *J. Parenter. Drug. Assoc.*, *33*, 257—272 (1979).
53. M. J. Akers, I. A. Attia, and K. E. Avis, Understanding and utilizing F_0 values, *Pharm. Tech.*, *2*, 31—35 (1978).
54. J. B. Selkon, P. R. Sisson, and H. R. Ingham, The use of spore strips for monitoring the sterilization of bottled fluids, *J. Hyg.* (Lond.), *83*, 121—125 (1979).
55. D. H. Dadd and G. M. Daley, Resistance of microorganisms to inactivation by gaseous ethylene oxide, *J. Appl. Bacteriol.*, *49*, 89—101 (1980).
56. P. M. Borick and J. A. Borick, Sterility of pharmaceuticals, cosmetics, and medical devices, *Quality Control in the Pharmaceutical Industry*, Volume 1 (M. S. Cooper, Ed.), Academic Press, New York, 1972, p. 17.
57. T. Myers and S. Chrai, Parenteral fundamentals: basic principles and applications of bioindicators, *J. Parenter. Drug. Assoc.*, *34*, 234—243 (1980).

58. R. A. Caputo and C. C. Mascoli, The design and use of biological indicators for sterilization cycle validation, *Med. Device Diagn.*, *2*, 23 (1980).

59. I. J. Pflug and T. E. Odlaug, *Syllabus for an Introductory Course in the Microbiology and Engineering of Sterilization Processes*, Environmental Sterilization Services, St. Paul, Minnesota, Aug. 1978.

60. R. A. Caputo, T. E. Odlaug, R. L. Wilkinson, and C. C. Mascoli, Biological validation of a steam-sterilized product by the fractional exposure method, *J. Parenter. Drug Assoc.*, *33*, 214—221 (1979).

61. Federal Standard No. 209B, Clean Room and Work Station Requirements, Controlled Environment, General Services Administration, Washington, D. C., Aug. 10, 1966.

62. W. Whitfield, *Contam. Contr.*, *3*, 16 (1964).

63. G. B. Phillips and W. S. Miller, Sterilization, in *Remington's Pharmaceutical Sciences*, 16th Edition, Mack Publishing, Easton, Pennsylvania, 1980, pp. 1399—1400.

64. Personal communication, K. E. Avis, College of Pharmacy, University of Tennessee Center for the Health Sciences, Memphis, Tennessee.

65. R. I. Gross, Laminar flow equipment performance and testing requirements, *Bull. Parenter. Drug Assoc.*, *30*, 143—151 (1976).

66. R. I. Gross, Testing of laminar flow equipment, *J. Parenter. Drug. Assoc.*, *32*, 174—181 (1978).

67. ASTM D2986-71, Standard method for evaluation of air assay media by the monodisperse DOP smoke test.

68. G. B. Phillips and R. S. Runkle, *Biomedical Applications of Laminar Airflow*, CRC Press, Cleveland, Ohio, 1973.

69. K. E. Avis, Parenteral preparations, in *Remington's Pharmaceutical Sciences*, 16th Edition, Mack Publishing, Easton, Pennsylvania, 1980, pp. 1470—1475.

70. R. R. Austin and S. W. Timmerman, *Design and Operation of Clean Rooms*, Business News Publishing, Detroit, Michigan, 1965.

71. R. P. Delmore and W. N. Thompson, A comparison of air-sampler efficiencies, *Med. Device Diagn.*, *3*, 45 (1981).

72. G. Kraidman, The microbiology of airborne contamination and air sampling, *Drug Cosmet. Ind.*, *116*, 40—45 (1975).

73. L. A. Dell, Aspects of microbiological monitoring for non-sterile and sterile manufacturing environments, *Pharm. Tech.*, *3*, 47—51 (1979).

74. F. A. DeVecchi, Training personnel to work in sterile environments, *Pharm. Tech.*, *2*, 41–44 (1978).

75. M. A. -F. Abdou, Determination of airborne microorganisms in a pharmaceutical plant using standard elective and selective culture media, *Pharm. Tech.*, *4*, 93–100 (1980).

76. K. L. Brier, C. J. Latiolais, P. J. Schneider et al., Effect of laminar air flow and clean-room dress on contamination rates of intravenous admixtures, *Amer. J. Hosp. Pharm.*, *38*, 1144–1147.

77. W. A. Gouvia and E. R. Anderson, Protecting our investment in sterile products, *Amer. J. Hosp. Pharm.*, *37*, 1311 (1980).

78. B. L. Green and W. Litsky, Evaluation of a closed system for sterility testing of parenterals, *Pharm. Tech.*, *3*, 72–77 (1979).

79. C. G. Mayhall, P. G. Pierpaoli, G. O. Hall, and R. B. Thomas, Evaluation of a device for monitoring sterility of injectable fluids, *Amer. J. Hosp. Pharm.*, *38*, 1148–1150 (1981).

80. L. M. Posey, R. E. Nutt, and P. D. Thomson, Comparison of two methods for detecting microbial contamination in intravenous fluids, *Amer. J. Hosp. Pharm.*, *38*, 659–662 (1981).

81. F. Condella, K. Eichelberger, L. C. Foote, and R. E. Griffin, Evaluation of two sterility testing methods for intravenous admixtures, *Hosp. Pharm.*, *15*, 305–310 (1980).

82. K. H. Hoffman, F. M. Smith, H. N. Godwin, L. C. Hogan, and D. Furtado, Evaluation of three methods for detecting bacterial contamination in intravenous solutions, *Amer. J. Hosp. Pharm.*, *39*, 1299–1302 (1982).

83. C. M. Miller, D. Furtado, F. M. Smith, H. N. Godwin, L. C. Hogan, and D. E. Letendre, Evaluation of three methods for detecting low-level bacterial contamination in intravenous solutions, *Amer. J. Hosp. Pharm.*, *39*, 1302–1305 (1982).

84. M. Pickett and L. Litsky, An effective alternative for testing antibiotic sterility, *Pharm. Tech.*, *5*, 63–68 (1981).

85. J. C. Lim, Technique of microbiological testing of in-use intravenous solutions and administration sets, *Amer. J. Hosp. Pharm.*, *36*, 1202–1204 (1979).

86. C. A. Rupp, C. A. Kikugawa, S. E. Kotabe et al., Quality control of small-volume sterile products, *Amer. J. Hosp. Pharm.*, *34*, 47–49 (1977).

87. S. P. Deniser and K. H. Ward, A rapid method for the detection of 59 bacterial contaminants in intravenous fluids using membrane filtration and epifluorescence microscopy, *J. Parenter. Sci. Tech.*, *37*, 156–158 (1983).

88. J. A. Rycroft and D. Moon, An in-production method for testing the sterility of infusion fluids, *J. Hyg. Camb.*, *74*, 17–25 (1975).

89. T. R. Rameshbabu and A. S. Arambulo, Early detection of microbial contamination in sterile solutions using an electronic counter, *Bull. Parenter. Drug Assoc.*, *30*, 80–87 (1976).

90. C. A. Bopp and I. K. Wachsmuth, Luciferase assay to detect bacterial contamination of intravenous fluids, *Amer. J. Hosp. Pharm.*, *38*, 1747–1750 (1981).

2
Pyrogen Testing

When injected into man in sufficient amounts, pyrogens will cause
a variety of adverse physiological responses (Table 2.1). The
most common or recognizable response is an increase in body temperature, from which the name "pyrogen" is derived (Greek
"pyro" = fire; "gen" = beginning). Pyrogenic responses rarely
are fatal unless the patient is very sick and the dose is very
large. Nevertheless, pyrogens are considered toxic substances
and should never be injected knowingly. Pyrogen contamination
of large-volume parenteral solutions is especially serious because
of the large amounts of fluid administered to people whose illnesses
must be of the severity to warrant the use of such large volumes.

Pyrogens come from microorganisms. All microbial forms produce pyrogen; however, the most potent pyrogen originates from
gram negative bacteria. The entity primarily involved in pyrogenic reactions in mammals is the lipopolysaccharide (LPS) from
the outer cell membranes of gram negative bacteria (1). Another
name for LPS is endotoxin. Although not entirely correct, the
names pyrogen, LPS, and endotoxin are routinely used inter-
changeably in parenteral circles. Figure 2.1 is a schematic representation of the three cell wall layers of a gram negative microorganism (1). The outer membrane shown in the figure is not
found in gram positive bacteria. This structure contains the LPS

TABLE 2.1   Adverse Physiological Effects of Pyrogens in Man

Primary

 1. Increase in body temperature
 2. Chilly sensation
 3. Cutaneous vasoconstriction
 4. Pupillary dilation
 5. Piloerection
 6. Decrease in respiration
 7. Rise in arterial blood pressure
 8. Nausea and malaise
 9. Severe diarrhea
10. Pain in the back and legs
11. Headache

Secondary

 1. Cutaneous vasodilation
 2. Hyperglycemia
 3. Sweating
 4. Fall in arterial blood pressure
 5. Involuntary urination and defecation
 6. Decreased gastric secretion and motility
 7. Penile erection
 8. Leucocytopenia, leucocytosis
 9. Hemorrhage and necrosis in tumors
10. Altered resistance to bacterial infections
11. Depletion of liver glycogen
12. Rise in blood ascorbic acid
13. Rise in blood non-protein nitrogen and uric acid
14. Decrease in plasma amino acids

---

moiety which interacts with the coagulable protein of the amebocytes of the horseshoe crab, a phenomenon from which evolved
the Limulus Amebocyte Lysate (LAL) test.

LPS, extracted and recovered as a colloidal suspension, may be
split by mild acid hydrolysis into lipid A and degraded polysac-
charides (2). Lipid A is composed of B-1, 6-glucosamine disac-
charide units with β-hydroxymyristic acid replacing one of the
amino hydrogens, and fatty acids replacing hydrogen in some of
the —OH groups (see Figure 2.2). Each two glucosamine units

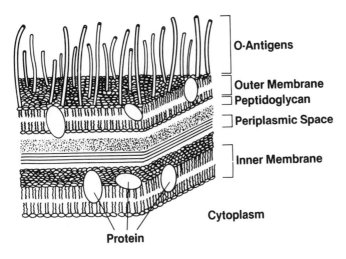

FIGURE 2.1   Schematic representation of the three cell wall layers of a gram-negative bacterium (From Ref. 1.)

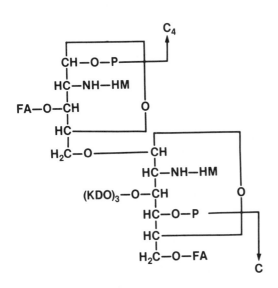

FIGURE 2.2   Structure of unit of Lipid A from Salmonella lipopolysaccharide.   KDO: 3-deoxy-D-mannooctulosonic acid; HM: β-hydroxymyristic acid; FA: other long chain fatty acids. (Reproduced in part from Ref. 2 and Rietschel et al., *Eur. J. Biochem.*, *28*, 166, 1972.)

are separated by two phosphate moieties forming a linear polymer (1). Lipid A alone lacks biologic activity, yet LPS is toxic, probably because polysaccharide increases the aqueous solubility of lipid A. Kennedi et al. (3) showed that when lipid A is separated from the polysaccharide component of endotoxin, it loses more than 99.9% of its pyrogenic activity in rabbits.

Freedom from pyrogenic contamination characterizes parenteral products in the same manner as sterility and freedom from particulate matter. Preventing the presence of pyrogens is much preferred over removing pyrogens in parenteral products. Preventing pyrogenic contamination primarily involves the use of ingredients, solvents, packaging materials, and processing equipment that have been depyrogenated initially, then employing correct and proper procedures during the entire manufacturing process to minimize the possibility of pyrogen development.

HISTORY

The pyrogenic response has been known since 1865 when it was reported that an injection of distilled water produced hyperthermia in dogs (4). Later, in 1876, the presence of a fever-producing substance, called "pyrogen" for the first time, was found in extracts of putrefying meat (5). Identification of the pyrogenic component from bacteria was attempted by Roussy in 1889 (6) and Centanni in 1894 (7), who determined that pyrogen was non-proteinaceous. Hort and Penfold (8) in 1911 made significant contributions in relating the production of fever and the administration of intravenous infusions. They also were the first to use rabbits as an animal model to study the pyrogenic response. They showed that the incidence of chills and fever following intravenous injection could be reduced markedly if freshly prepared distilled water was used as the injection solvent. Investigators (9,10) related fever production in rabbits with the injection of bacterial culture extracts and showed that sterile solutions free from endotoxins did not cause the febrile response. Pyrogenicity seemed to be related to the gram-stain reaction; gram negative organisms produced a pyrogenic response while gram positive organisms did not. Additionally, bacterial pyrogens were not destroyed by autoclaving or removed by filtration.

It is interesting to note that while the medical significance of pyrogen was recognized during these years, it was not until 1923 that Florence Seibert (11,12) recommended that all pharmaceuticals be tested for pyrogens. Seibert's carefully controlled experiments confirmed Hort and Penfold's results using the rabbit as the animal model for detecting the presence of pyrogens in injectables. Seibert also demonstrated conclusively that pyrogens originate from water-borne organisms, are heat resistant and filterable, and can be eliminated in water by distillation. Rademacher (13) substantiated Seibert's results and presented instructions for the preparation of pyrogen-free parenteral solutions. CoTui and Schrift (14) reported that the pyrogen-producing characteristics of microorganisms depend on the type of organism and that bacterial pyrogens are related to lipopolysaccharides.

The pyrogen test became an official quality control test for parenterals in 1942 in the United States Pharmacopeia (USP) 12th edition. Later, in 1945, the Code of Federal Regulations* required antibiotics to be tested for pyrogens. Despite the advances in parenteral science and technology over the past 40 years, the rabbit pyrogen test methodology officially recognized in compendial standards has remained essentially unchanged.

SPECIFIC REQUIREMENTS OF THE
USP RABBIT PYROGEN TEST

Since its inception in the USP in 1942, the rabbit pyrogen test has remained essentially unchanged. Thus, the content of this section will follow closely both the specifications written in the 21st edition of the USP (15) and the excellent review article written in 1973 by Personeus (16).

General Description of the USP Pyrogen Test

The following paragraph is quoted directly from the USP, under the section on pyrogen testing:

The pyrogen test is designed to limit to an acceptable level the risks of febrile reaction in the patient to the administration, by injection, of the product concerned. The test involves measuring the rise in temperature of rabbits following the intravenous injection of a test solution and is designed for products that can be tolerated by the test rabbit in a dose not to exceed

---

*CFR Title 21, Section 610.13 for biologicals and Sections 436.31 and 436.32 for antibiotics.

10 ml per kg injected intravenously within a period of not more than 10 minutes. For products that require preliminary preparation or are subject to special conditions of administration, follow the additional directions given in the individual monograph or, in the case of antibiotics or biologics, the additional directions given in the federal regulations.

Apparatus and Diluents

All apparatuses—glassware, containers, syringes, needles, etc.—and all diluents used in performing the pyrogen test must themselves be free from pyrogenic contamination. Heat-durable items such as glass and stainless steel can be depyrogenated by exposure to dry heat cycles at temperatures greater than 250°C for at least 30 minutes. Diluents and solutions for washing and rinsing of devices are to be pyrogen free. Commercially available sterile and pyrogen-free solution products usually are employed.

To ensure the lack of pyrogenicity with the various materials used in conducting the pyrogen test, negative controls should be performed with each test. Negative controls utilize the diluent rather than the product sample as the injection, with the diluent being exposed to the same procedure and materials as the product sample. The use of negative controls with each pyrogen test is not standard practice because of prior knowledge and assurance that materials used in the test are non-pyrogenic.

Temperature Recording

The USP states the following:

Use an accurate temperature-sensing device such as a clinical thermometer, or thermistor probes or similar probes that have been calibrated to assure an accuracy of ±0.1°C and have been tested to determine that a maximum reading is reached in less than 5 minutes. Insert the temperature-sensing probe into the rectum of the test rabbit to a depth of not less than 7.5 cm, and, after a period of time not less than that previously determined as sufficient, record the rabbit's body temperature.

Thermocouples connected to electronic recording devices are almost exclusively used today for measuring temperature rectally in rabbits. A thermocouple contains two dissimilar electrical conductor wires joined at one end to form a measuring junction which produces a thermal electromotive force (EMF). There exist several

TABLE 2.2   Commonly Used Thermocouple Types

Type B	Platinum-30 percent rhodium (+) versus platinum-6 percent rhodium (-)
Type E	Nickel-10 percent chromium (+) versus constantan (-)
Type J	Iron (+) versus constantan (-)
Type K	Nickel-10 percent chromium (+) versus Nickel-5 percent (-)
Type R	Platinum-13 percent rhodium (+) versus platinum (-)
Type S	Platinum-10 percent rhodium (+) versus platinum (-)
Type T	Copper (+) versus constantan (-)

thermocouple types, each having a defined EMF-temperature relationship. For example, at a temperature of 100°F, a type T (copper-constantan) thermocouple will generate an EMF of 1.518 millivolts. Common thermocouple types are listed in Table 2.2. Typical thermocouples are composed of three parts as shown in Figure 2.3. The two dissimilar wires are supported by an electrical insulator, either hard-fired ceramic or non-ceramic materials such as Teflon, polyvinyl chloride, fiber glass, fibrous silica, or asbestos. The outer sheath can be composed from a variety of materials, most commonly stainless steel, Teflon, and various elemental metals (platinum, copper, and aluminum).

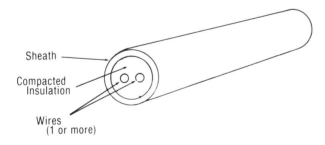

Sheath

Compacted
Insulation

Wires
(1 or more)

FIGURE 2.3   Composition of a typical thermocouple used in rabbit pyrogen testing. (Courtesy of the American Society for Testing and Materials, Philadelphia, Pennsylvania.)

Thermocouples must be accurately calibrated against National Bureau of Standards (NBS) traceable standard constant temperature baths. Accuracy of thermocouple temperature measurement can never exceed the accuracy of the thermocouple reference. Reference instrumentation should include both an ice point reference bath and an elevated temperature reference bath. These calibration baths initially should be calibrated against an electronic monitor incorporating an NBS-traceable standard resistor with an accurate and constant source of current. Once the baths are calibrated, the thermocouples can be placed in the wells of the baths and temperature accuracy determined. The accuracy of the thermocouples must be ±0.1°C of the calibration bath temperature or should not be used in pyrogen testing.

Rabbit body temperature data are recorded electronically by instruments such as those seen in Figure 2.4. Electronic temperature recorders usually can monitor over 100 rabbits simultaneously. Any variation in room temperature must be compensated by built-in calibration capability of the recorder. Proper maintenance and repair of recording devices must be accomplished.

Computerized equipment are now available for automatic temperature recording during pyrogen testing. A recent description of computerized temperature recording in pyrogen testing was published by Joubert (17).

Test Animals

Rabbits are used as pyrogen test models because they physiologically respond similarly to pyrogens as do human beings. Griesman and Hornick (18) showed that rabbits and humans respond identically on a nanogram per kilogram basis to pyrogenic quantities of endotoxin.

Quoting from the USP:

Use healthy, mature rabbits. House the rabbits individually in an area of uniform temperature between 20°C and 23°C and free from disturbances likely to excite them. The temperature varies not more than ±3°C from the selected temperature. Before using a rabbit for the first time in a pyrogen test, condition it not more than seven days before use by a sham test that includes all of the steps as directed under Procedure except injection. Do not use a rabbit for pyrogen testing more frequently than once every 48 hours, nor prior to 2 weeks following a maximum rise of its temperature of 0.6°C or more while being subjected to the pyrogen test or following its having been given a test specimen that was adjudged pyrogenic.

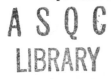

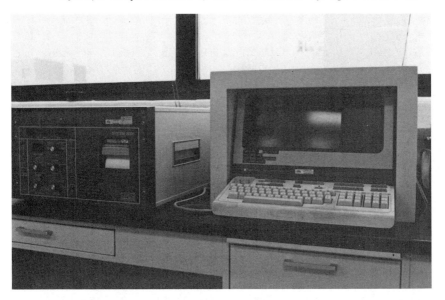

FIGURE 2.4   Electronic thermal recording instruments used to monitor rabbit body temperatures during the pyrogen test.

Several strains of rabbits are acceptable as test animals for the pyrogen test. Key factors in selecting rabbits are the animal breeder, rabbit resistance to disease, sufficient size for ease of handling, large ears, and rate of weight gain. The albino rabbit is the most widely used rabbit, particularly strains from New Zealand and Belgium.

It is essential that the rabbit colony be treated with utmost care. The environment in which the rabbits are housed must be strictly controlled with respect to temperature, humidity, lighting, and potential contamination of air, surfaces, and feed. Any new shipment of rabbits should be quarantined and monitored for one to two weeks following receipt of the shipment for presence of illness and/or disease.

Rabbits must be trained to adjust and adapt to their new environment in the pyrogen testing laboratory. Methods applied have been reviewed by Personeus (16). Rabbits must become accustomed to being restrained in their cages and being handled both in the rectal insertion of the thermocouple and the injection of the test product.

The normal basal body temperature of rabbits ranges between 38.9 and 39.8°C (102.0-103.6°F). Rabbit baseline temperature is established by measuring rectal temperature during the conductance of several "sham" tests (following the entire pyrogen test procedure using pyrogen-free sodium chloride solution as the injection sample). Such tests should be, but rarely are, conducted over a period of several weeks. Temperature variances will occur in untrained rabbits, but upon training temperature variation will diminish to an acceptable range of ±0.2°C. The normal temperature range of a rabbit may shift with time, requiring the re-establishment of the true normal body temperature.

Rabbits may become tolerant to pyrogenic activity after repeated injections of endotoxin (19-21). It is for this reason that a rabbit showing a rise of its body temperature of 0.6°C or more during a pyrogen test cannot be used again as a pyrogen test animal for at least two weeks.

Test Procedures

The USP procedure recommended for performing the pyrogen test is reprinted as follows:

Perform the test in a separate area designated solely for pyrogen testing and under environmental conditions similar to those under which the animals are housed and free from disturbances likely to excite them. Withhold all food from the rabbits used during the period of the test. Access to water is allowed at all times, but may be restricted during the test. If rectal temperature-measuring probes remain inserted throughout the testing period, restrain the rabbits with light-fitting stocks that allow the rabbits to assume a natural resting posture. Not more than 30 minutes prior to the injection of the test dose, determine the "control temperature" of each rabbit. This is the base for the determination of any temperature increase resulting from the injection of a test solution. In any one group of test rabbits, use only those rabbits whose control temperatures do not vary by more than 1 degree from each other, and do not use any rabbit having a temperature exceeding 39.8°C.

Unless otherwise specified in the individual monograph, inject into an ear vein of each of three rabbits 10 ml of the test solution per kg of body weight, completing each injection within 10 minutes after the start of administration. The test solution is either the product, constituted if necessary as directed in the labeling, or the material under test treated as directed in the

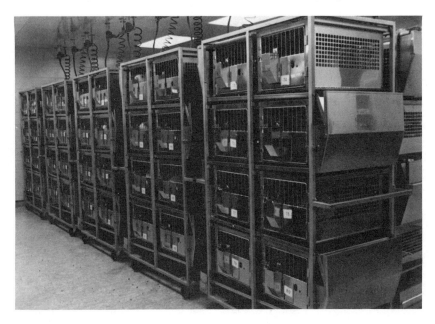

FIGURE 2.5   Housing of pyrogen test rabbits in clean, individual cages.

individual monograph and injected in the dose specified therein. For pyrogen testing of devices or injection assemblies, use washings or rinsings of the surfaces that come in contact with the parenterally-administered material or with the injection site or internal tissues of the patient. [For example, the third supplement of the USP XX/NF XV (p. 300) requires that 40 ml of sterile, pyrogen-free saline, TS as a flow rate of approximately 10 ml per minute are to be passed through the tubing of each of 10 transfusion of infusion assemblies.] Assure that all test solutions are protected from contamination. Perform the injection after warming the test solution to a temperature of 37 ± 2°C. Record the temperature at 1, 2, and 3 hours subsequent to the injection.

Rabbits belong in a facility that is temperature-controlled, e.g., 70 ± 5°F. Housing should be individual cages designed to maintain cleanliness (see Figure 2.5). Cage design should conform to standards established by the American Association of Accreditation of Laboratory Animal Care (AAALAC).

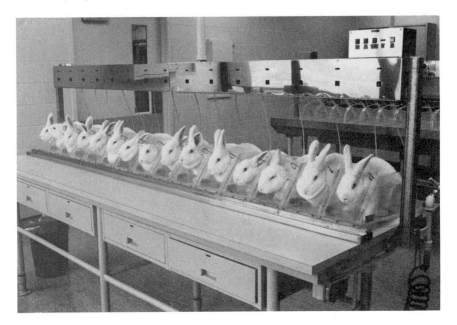

FIGURE 2.6   Rabbits situated in individual restraining boxes.

The facility has two basic rooms. One room houses the rabbits
between tests while the other room is used only for actual pyrogen
testing. Rabbits in restraining boxes (see Figure 2.6) are trans-
ported on carts or wagons from the holding room into the testing
room. The two rooms should have a door between them which is
closed during the pyrogen testing period. Environmental conditions in the two rooms should be identical.

Noise represents a major problem in maintaining and using rabbits for pyrogen testing. The room in which the tests are conducted should be as free from noise and activity as possible.
Anything that causes excitement in the rabbit potentially can produce a 0.2-1.0°C rise in body temperature which may not return
to normal for 60-90 minutes.

During the pyrogen test, which could last four to six hours,
the rabbits should be restrained with a minimum of discomfort.
Restraint should be confined to the neck and head of the rabbit
to facilitate the test dose injection into the ear vein and to permit
the rabbit comfortable movement of its legs and back. Examples
of modern restraining boxes are shown in Figures 2.6 and 2.7.

Rabbits that have been adequately trained, are healthy, and exhibit stable body temperatures are selected for the pyrogen test. The animals are weighed and placed in their restraining boxes. Thermocouples (see Figure 2.7) are inserted in the rectum to a depth of not less than 7.5 cm. Following a 30-45 minute acclimation period, the control temperature reading of the rabbit is recorded. Within 30 minutes of the recording of the control temperature, the test dose should be administered.

Dose administration is accomplished using a sterile syringe and 20-23 gauge needle. The size of syringe will depend on the dose volume. The USP requires a dose of 10 ml per kg body weight unless otherwise specified in the individual monograph. For example, Phytonadione Injection, USP, pyrogen test dose is 2 ml per kg while Protamine Sulfate Injection, USP requires only 0.5 ml per kg containing 10 mg per ml. Some injectable monographs specify the pyrogen test dose on a weight-weight basis, e.g., the dose of Diazepam Injection, USP is 0.25 mg per kg.

The test solution must be warmed to 37°C prior to injection. The ear vein is swabbed with alcohol (70%), which not only disinfects

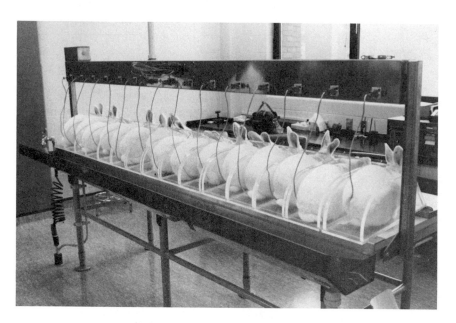

FIGURE 2.7   Rear view of rabbits in restraining boxes.

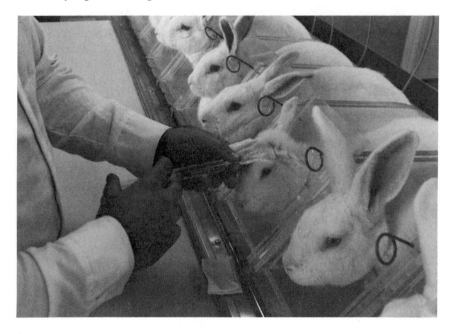

FIGURE 2.8   Injection of pyrogen test sample into ear vein of rabbit.

but also improves visibility of the vein.   Vein longevity can be preserved by employing correct technique in making the injection. A suggested procedure is the following:

1. Rest the ear against the fingers of the left hand and hold the ear down with the thumb (see Figure 2.8).
2. Introduce the needle with the bevel edge upward near the tip of the ear vein.
3. Slowly inject a small amount of sample to determine if the needle is within the vein lumen.   If not, a bubble will form or back pressure will be felt.   Withdrawing the needle slightly and moving it forward again should place it in proper position.
4. Maintain steady pressure on the syringe plunger and complete the injection within 10 minutes.   Usually the time duration for infusion is much less than 10 minutes.
5. Withdraw the needle and apply pressure with the thumb at the site of injection to retard bleeding and scarring.

Rectal temperatures are recorded at one, two, and three hours subsequent to the injection. During the test period rabbits and equipment should be checked periodically. Occasionally a rabbit may experience rectal bleeding, irritation, or leg or back discomfort. Thermocouple wires might break or the electronic thermal recorders may malfunction. Immediate action should be taken in any of these situations.

Mazur and McKendrick (22) have reported on the automated pyrogen test system used by McGaw Laboratories. The system manages all phases of the pyrogen test, including setting up the test, acquiring and recording animal temperature data, calculating test results, and issuing release reports. Today most modern pyrogen testing laboratories utilize similar computer technology.

Test Interpretation—USP

The solution may be judged non-pyrogenic if (a) no single rabbit shows a rise in temperature of 0.6°C or greater above its control temperature, and (b) the sum of three individual maximum temperature increases over the three-hour test period does not exceed 1.4°C. If either of these two conditions is not met, the test must proceed to a second stage. In the second stage, five additional rabbits are given a new preparation of the same test sample as the original three rabbits. The solution may be judged non-pyrogenic if (a) not more than three of the eight rabbits showed individual temperature rises of 0.6°C or more and (b) the sum of all eight individual maximum temperature increases does not exceed 3.7°C.

The United States Public Health Requirements for Biological Products, Part 73, judge a solution to be pyrogenic if at least half of the rabbits tested show a temperature rise of 0.6°C or more, or if the average temperature rise of all rabbits is 0.5°C or more.

The British Pharmacopoeia (23) pyrogen test employs a sliding scale based on three rabbits and additional groups of three rabbits, if required, for a total of 12 rabbits. This scale is shown in Table 2.3 with the USP test included for comparison.

Limitations of the USP Rabbit Pyrogen Test

The USP rabbit pyrogen suffers from several limitations which established the opportunity for the *Limulus* Amebocyte Lysate test as a possible alternative for the rabbit test as an official pyrogen test procedure.

TABLE 2.3 Comparison of United States Pharmacopeial (USP) and British Pharmacopoeial (BP) Pyrogen Tests Requirements

Number of rabbits	Maximum total peak response (°C) to pass the test		Minimum total peak response (°C) to fail the test	
	USP	BP	USP	BP
3	1.4	1.15	1.4	2.65
6	–	2.80	–	4.30
8	3.7	–	3.7	–
9	–	4.45	–	5.95
12	–	6.60	–	6.60

In Vivo Model

A test method that uses a living animal as its model certainly must submit to a number of problems offered by biological systems. Variability in biological systems poses a great problem. No two rabbits will possess exactly the same body temperature or respond identically to the same pyrogenic sample. Rabbits are extremely sensitive and vulnerable to their environment. This translates into an expensive proposition in terms of facilities, control of the environment, and training of the animal.

Pyrogen testing of rabbits is not only expensive but also laborious. Several hours are consumed in performing the pyrogen test including a great amount of preliminary effort in preparing the animals. Rabbits must be fed and watered properly, cages cleaned to prevent disease, and time spent in training the animals to adapt to the conditions of the pyrogen testing facility and the test itself.

Rabbit Sensitivity to Pyrogens

The pyrogenic response in rabbits is dose dependent. The greater the amount of pyrogen injected per kg body weight, the greater the temperature increase in rabbits. This is demonstrated in Table 2.4, taken from a report by Mascoli and Weary (24).

A collaborative study initiated under the auspices of the Health Industry Manufacturers Association (HIMA) demonstrated that rabbits from 12 laboratories consistently failed (pyrogenic) the

TABLE 2.4 Eight Rabbit Pyrogen Test Results in Saline with *E. coli* 055:BS Using 3–5 Kg Rabbits

E. coli endotoxin concentration (ng/ml)	Volume solution injected (ml/kg)	USP total temperature increase (°C)	Mean temperature increase (°C)	Standard deviation (°C)	Coefficient of variation (%)
3.125	1.0	7.80[c]	0.975	0.246	25.2
1.56	1.0	4.75[c]	0.594	0.218	36.7
1.00	1.0	3.70[c]	0.462	0.158	34.2
0.78	1.0	1.40	0.144	0.208	144.4
0.39	1.0	1.00	0.088	0.187	212.5
0.195	1.0	1.20	0.150	0.065	43.3

[a]Negative rabbit temperature values were excluded from total temperature increase determinations according to USP.
[b]Negative rabbit temperature values were included in the determinations of means and standard deviations to properly reflect total variability.
[c]Fail USP test criteria of 3.7° total increase.
Source: Ref. 24.

test at $\geqslant 1.0$ ng per ml doses (10 ml/kg of 10 ng/kg endotoxin) of *E. coli* 055:B5 endotoxin, and all colonies passed (no pyrogenicity) at the 0.156 ng/kg dose (or 0.0156 ng/ml using a 10 ml/kg dose) (25). The same study reported that the "average" rabbit colony will attain a 50% pass/fail rate with 95% confidence at an endotoxin level above 0.098 ng/ml (10 ml/kg dose). The LAL test generally will detect endotoxin levels of 0.025 ng/ml or less. Thus, the rabbit test is less sensitive to endotoxin than the LAL test is.

Rabbit-to-rabbit variation in response to the same lot of pyrogenic solution has been shown by Mascoli and Weary (24). As seen in Table 2.4, the standard deviations and coefficient of variation values are rather high among eight rabbits administered identical doses of endotoxin. The HIMA study reported that out of 12 laboratories conducting rabbit pyrogen tests, four passed a level of 2.5 ng endotoxin per kg level (25).

Sensitivity of the rabbit bioassay for endotoxin appears to fall in the range of 1 to 10 ng/kg (18,26). Greisman and Hornick (18) found that the threshold pyrogenic dose of *E. coli* endotoxin for both rabbits and humans is 1.0 ng/kg of body weight. This holds true regardless of the volume of pyrogenic solution administered because of the dose (rather than concentration) dependency of the rabbit response to pyrogen.

Rabbit sensitivity to endotoxin varies with the time of day (circadian) and time of year (cirannual) (27). The greatest rise in temperature for any given dose of endotoxin occurred in the afternoon while the least rise occurred at midnight. At midnight the greatest sensitivity was seen at the end of October while the least was seen at the end of April. However, this was opposite at 10:00 a.m. Although not practical at all, it was suggested in this report that a rabbit colony be tested for its threshold sensitivity at the beginning of each month and at the hours when products would be tested normally. Thus, seasonal variability in sensitivity may be controlled.

Interferences of the Rabbit Pyrogen Test

Many products administered parenterally cannot be tested for pyrogens with the rabbit test because of interferences they create in the rabbit response to pyrogens, if they are present in the product. Any product having a pyretic side effect, such as the the prostaglandins and the cancer chemotherapeutic agents, will interfere with the rabbit response. Several products are inherently toxic to the rabbit (see Table 2.5) and must be diluted to

TABLE 2.5 Examples of Drugs and Drug Products
not Suitable for Testing by the USP Pyrogen Test

1. Most cancer chemotherapeutic agents
2. Most anesthetics, muscle relaxants, and sedatives
3. Sterile Betamethasone Sodium Phosphate Solution
4. Chlorpheniramine injection
5. Magnesium sulfate
6. Metocurine iodide injection
7. Perphenazine
8. Thiopental sodium for injection

concentrations far below the pharmacologically effective dose of
the drug.

Despite these major limitations and the insurgence today of the
Limulus Amebocyte Lysate (LAL) test, it must not be forgotten
that the USP rabbit pyrogen test for decades has nobly served as
a sufficiently sensitive test for pyrogens and has helped to eliminate pyrogenic contamination from drugs reaching the market-
place.

THE LAL TEST

History and Background

Credit for discovering the interaction between endotoxin and the
amebocyte lysate of the horseshoe crab, *Limulus polyphemus*,
belongs to Levin and Bang (28). Basing their work upon earlier
research by Bang (29), these workers were involved in the study
of clotting mechanisms of the blood of lobsters, fish, and crabs.
Autopsies of dead horseshoe crabs revealed intravascular coagulation. The clotted blood was cultured and found to contain gram
negative bacteria such as *E. coli* and *Pseudomonas*. Further
tests showed that amebocyte cells of the horseshoe crab's blood
were extremely sensitive to the presence of endotoxin, the toxic
substance liberated by the disintegration of bacterial cells. The
substance in the amebocytes responsible for reacting with endotoxin is known to be a clottable protein, to be discussed in the
following section, "LAL Reaction Mechanism." In lysing the amebocyte cells by osmotic effects, a most sensitive biochemical indicator of the presence of endotoxin was produced, hence the name
Limulus Amebocyte Lysate test.

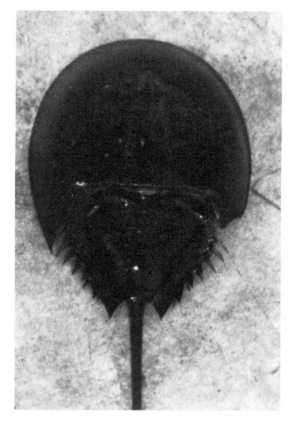

FIGURE 2.9 *Limulus polyphemus,* the source of Limulus amebocyte lysate reagent.

Limulus polyphemus (see Figure 2.9) is found only at specific
locations along the east coast of North America and the coasts
along Southeast Asia. The hearts of mature crabs are punctured
and bled to collect the circulating amebocyte blood cells. Carefully performed, this procedure is not fatal to the crab, and upon
proper restoration, the crab can be used again. Since amebocytes
act as activators of the coagulation mechanism in the crab, an
anti-aggregating agent must be added to inhibit aggregation.
N-ethylmaleimade is the most commonly used anti-aggregant.

Amebocyte cells are collected and washed by centrifugation,
and lysed using distilled water. Lysing can also be done with

ultrasound, freezing and thawing, and grinding in a glass tissue homogenizer (30). After lysing, the suspension is cleared of debris by centrifugation and the supernate is lyophilized. Lyophilization is necessary for stability purposes. LAL reagent is extremely sensitive to heat and even in the lyophilized state must be stored in the freezer (31). Upon reconstitution LAL has a shelf life of one month's storage at freezing conditions.

The LAL test for pyrogens in parenterals was first applied by Cooper et al. (32). The LAL test was found to be more sensitive than the rabbit pyrogen test in the testing of radioactive drug products. Mallinckrodt, Inc., established the first successful, large-scale production facility for LAL in Chincoteague, Virginia, in 1971 (33).

On January 12, 1973 (Federal Register 38:1404), the FDA stated that LAL was a biological product, thus subject to licensing under Section 351 of the Public Health Service Act. Specifications concerning the purity and potency of LAL were proposed by the FDA Bureau of Biologics later that year (September 18, 1973; 38 FR 26130). In the ensuing years, available data on and experience with the LAL test accumulated with the primary use of the test being an in-process endotoxin test. Finally, the FDA announced conditions under which the LAL test could be used as an end-product test for licensed biological products and medical devices (November 4, 1977; 42 FR 57749). This was followed by a draft guideline published by the Office of Medical Devices for using the LAL test for medical devices exclusively (March 20, 1979).

In the Federal Register of January 18, 1980 (45 FR 3668), the FDS published a notice announcing the availability of a draft guideline describing the conditions for validating the LAL test before using it as a final end-product endotoxin test for human and veterinary injectable drug products. Comments on the two draft guidelines (March, 1979 and January, 1980) resulted in a single draft guideline for validation of the LAL test as an end-product endotoxin test for human and animal parenteral drugs, biological products, and medical devices published on February 2, 1983 and announced on March 29, 1983 (48 FR 13098). Specific details of this draft are identified in later sections of this chapter.

Until 1977, the Bureau of Biologics prepared its own lysate. Since then the Bureau has found it more economical to purchase licensed lysate from one of several licensed manufacturers. The specifications required by the FDA before purchasing a lot of LAL are summarized in Table 2.6 (34).

TABLE 2.6 Summary of FDA Standards Governing the Manufacture of Limulus Amebocyte Lysate Reagent

---

1. Use of United States Standard Endotoxin for determining the sensitivity of LAL.

2. Use of United States Reference LAL for establishing the potency of LAL.

3. Calculation of potency of each lot of LAL and the U.S. Reference LAL using the U.S. Standard Endotoxin.

    a. Test a minimum of 20 to a maximum of 28 vials per each drying chamber.
    b. The 99% fiducial upper limit of the standard deviation of the log ratio of reference and test lysates for 20 vials can be no greater than 0.73.

4. General requirements.

    a. Handle horseshoe crabs in a manner to enable them to be returned alive to their natural environment after a single collection of blood.
    b. Perform sterility test on bulk lot and on each filling.
    c. Run negative control tests of lysate.
    d. Test for residual moisture.

5. Various labeling requirements.

6. Appropriate number of samples (not fewer than 28 vials) and documentation of manufacture of each filling, dates of testing, and results of all tests must be submitted to Director, Bureau of Biologics, FDA.

Source: Ref. 34.

LAL Reaction Mechanism

Elucidation of the endotoxin-LAL reaction has resulted primarily from the work by Liu et al. (35), Takagi et al. (36), and Mosesson et al. (37). Combining the results of these researchers' efforts produces the following proposed reaction:

1. Endotoxin or a suitably prepared lipid-A derivative of endotoxin activates a proenzyme of LAL having a molecular weight of 150,000.

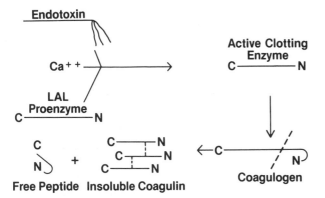

FIGURE 2.10   Schematic representation of the LAL reaction
mechanism. (From Ref. 39.)

2. Activation also depends on the presence of divalent metal
    cations such as calcium, manganese, or magnesium. It has
    been shown that the sensitivity of the LAL assay for endo-
    toxin detection can be increased 10 to 30 times by using
    LAL reagent containing 50 mM magnesium (38).
3. The activated proenzyme, related to the serine protease
    class containing such enzymes as thrombin, trypsin, and
    factor Xa, subsequently reacts with a lower molecular weight
    protein fraction (MW = 19,000–25,000) contained also in the
    LAL substance.
4. The lower molecular weight fraction, called coagulogen, is
    cleaved by the proenzyme into a soluble and insoluble sub-
    unit. The insoluble sub-unit appears as a solid clot, a
    precipitate, or a turbid solution, depending on the amount
    of insoluble coagulogen by-product formed.

Therefore, the coagulation reaction requires three factors in
addition to endotoxin. These three factors—a clotting enzyme,
clottable protein (coagulogen), and certain divalent cations—are
found in the LAL reagent. A schematic representation of the LAL
reaction mechanism is found in Figure 2.10 (39).

LAL Test Procedure

Cooper (40) first described the methods and materials required to
perform correctly the LAL test for pyrogen. While the LAL test

is a relatively simple procedure, especially when compared with the USP rabbit test, certain specific conditions must be met. These include:

1. All materials that will come into contact with the LAL reagent or test sample must be thoroughly cleaned and depyrogenated.
2. The reaction temperature cannot be outside the range of 36–38°C.
3. The pH of the reaction mixture must be within the range of pH 5–7.
4. The reaction time should be no longer than one hour.
5. Each test must be accompanied by positive and negative controls.

The basic procedure of the LAL test is the combination of 0.1 ml test sample with 0.1 ml LAL reagent. After one hour incubation at 37°C, the mixture is analyzed for the presence of a gel clot. The LAL test is positive, indicating the presence of endotoxin, if the gel clot maintains its integrity after slow inversion of the test tube containing the mixture (see Figure 2.11).

Complete instructions for conducting the LAL test are found in inserts supplied with LAL test kits from commercial manufacturers. The USP (21st edition) also contains instructions for using the LAL test to estimate the concentration of bacterial endotoxins in sample materials. These instructions will be summarized with commentary below:

Preliminary

1. Strict aseptic technique must be used to avoid microbial contamination while conducting the test.
2. All containers and equipment used must be pyrogen-free. Heating at 250°C or above for at least 60 minutes should depyrogenate these items.
3. All glassware should be washed with detergent prior to dry heat depyrogenation. If detergent is not completely rinsed away it will interfere with the reaction and cause a false negative result.
4. Abide by all precautions in reconstituting and storing the test reagents. Do not store diluted endotoxin used to determine LAL sensitivity because of loss of activity by adsorption to glass surfaces. The normal shelf life for LAL reagent is four weeks at freezing temperatures after reconstitution.

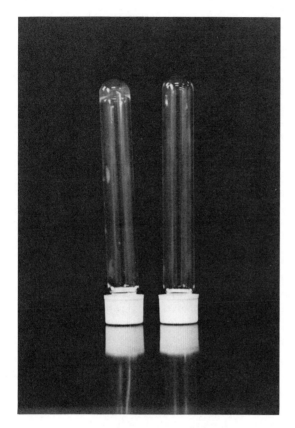

FIGURE 2.11   Example of a positive LAL test result showing an intact gel at the top of the inverted test tube on the left.

Standards

This topic can be confusing because the endotoxin standard used for drugs and biologicals is different from the standard used for medical devices. Also, the terms used for expressing endotoxin limits for drugs and devices are different, as will be discussed in the section "Endotoxin Limits in Parenteral Articles."

For drug and biological products, the endotoxin standard is called the U.S. Standard Endotoxin or the USP Reference Endotoxin (RSE). The first RSE lot was designated as Lot EC-2 and had a defined activity of one Endotoxin Unit (EU)* in 0.2 nanograms (ng) of the standard (41). The current RSE is Lot EC-5. One vial of EC-5 RSE contains 10,000 EUs.

For medical devices the endotoxin standard is Difco *E. coli* 055:B5 endotoxin. The Office of Medical Devices selected this endotoxin lot as its standard after a collaborative study with the medical device industry (see page 129 for details of this study). It is anticipated that when the device industry gains sufficient experience with the RSE, this will become the new standard for devices. At that time the Difco *E. coli* 055:B5 lot will become a Control Standard Endotoxin (CSE).

A CSE is an endotoxin preparation other than the reference standard endotoxin that has been standardized against the reference standard. CSE lots may be used in the place of the reference standard in laboratories conducting LAL tests.

If a manufacturer chooses to use a control standard endotoxin, the CSE will have to be standardized against the RSE. The following is an example of a procedure to determine the relationship of the CSE to the RSE (42):

At least four samples (vials) for the lot of CSE should be assayed. State in mg/ml and endpoint for the CSE and in EU/ml of the RSE. The values obtained should be the geometric mean of the endpoints using a minimum of four replicates. For example, if the LAL endpoints for the RSE and CSE were

CSE = 0.018 ng/ml

RSE = 0.3 EU/ml

then the amount of EUs per ng of CSE calculates to be

$$\frac{RSE}{CSE} = \frac{0.3 \text{ EU/ml}}{0.018 \text{ ng/ml}} = 16.6 \text{ EU/ng}$$

---

*It has become accepted practice to use Endotoxin Units (EU) as the more desirable expression of endotoxin strength than weight or concentration terms. The use of EU will allow any endotoxin type or lot to be used as a reference lot because its activity can always be related to the original U.S. Reference Standard lot. This chapter will use the EU term as much as possible, but most literature references cited will use the weight or concentration terms as reported in the published articles.

This indicates that 0.018 ng of CSE is equal to 0.3 EU of the RSE. Thus, the CSE contains 16.6 EU/ng.

Validation of the LAL Test

To validate the use of the LAL test for any application requires two determinations: (a) lysate sensitivity and (b) inhibition or enhancement properties of the product on the LAL-endotoxin interaction. Since validation requirements for LAL testing of drugs and biologicals differ somewhat from that for devices, these two product types will be covered separately.

Drugs and biological products

The LAL reagent used must have a confirmed potency (sensitivity). This is achieved by combining the particular reagent with a series of concentrations of RSE or CSE endotoxin bracketing the stated sensitivity (EU/ml) of the LAL reagent. Use four replicates per concentration of endotoxin. The series of endotoxin concentrations are prepared by twofold dilutions of the RSE or CSE endotoxin using LAL-negative water for injection. Following incubation and endpoint determination (manual or instrumental), the sensitivity of the LAL reagent will be confirmed if the test results are positive to within one twofold dilution of the stated label potency.

Inhibition/enhancement testing must be performed on undiluted drug products or diluted drug products not exceeding the minimum valid dilution value (see Table 2.7) (42). The product is spiked with various known amounts of RSE (or CSE), bracketing the sensitivity of the lysate used, using four replicate reaction tubes per level of endotoxin. The same number of tubes are used for drug product containing no added endotoxin and for control water for injection samples also spiked with various known amounts of RSE or CSE. The LAL test procedure is carried out manually or instrumentally. The end points (E in units per ml) are then observed and recorded for all replicate samples.

The end points are determined followed by computation of the geometric mean of these end points. Geometric mean is

$$\frac{\leq E \text{ (endpoints)}}{f \text{ (number of replicates)}}$$

and this mean is calculated for the control and test samples. An illustration is given in Table 2.8 (39). The geometric means of

TABLE 2.7 Examples of Minimum Valid Concentration (MVC) and Minimum Valid Dilution (MVD) Calculations

---

MVC Determination

$$MVC = \frac{\lambda M}{K}$$

λ = Sensitivity of LAL reagent in EU/ml

M = Rabbit dose or maximum human dose/kg

K = 5.0 EU/kg (0.2 EU/kg for intrathecal drugs)

If LAL sensitivity (λ) was 0.065 EU/ml, and the maximum human dose were 25 mg/kg, then the MCV would be:

$$MVC = \frac{0.065 \text{ EU/ml} \times 25 \text{ mg/kg}}{5.0 \text{ EU/kg}} = 0.325 \text{ mg/ml}$$

If this dose were to be given intrathecally, the denominator would be 0.2 EU/kg.

MVD Determination

$$MVD = \frac{\text{Potency of product}}{\text{MVC}}$$

If the potency of a product were 20 mg/ml, the MVD would be:

$$MVD = \frac{20 \text{ mg/ml}}{0.325 \text{ mg/ml}} = 1:61.5$$

Therefore, this product can be diluted to 61.5 times its original volume and still be able to detect the lower endotoxin concentration limit by the LAL test.

Source: Ref. 42.

TABLE 2.8   Example of Geometric Mean Determination for a
Small-Volume Parenteral Product Undergoing LAL Testing for
Endotoxin[a]

Replicates (f)		Gel endpoint results for specimen dilutions			Endpoint dilution factors (E)
	Unity	0.5	0.25	0.125	
1	+	+	+	−	0.25
2	+	+	−	−	0.5
3	+	+	−	−	0.5
4	+	+	+	−	0.25
5	+	+	−	−	0.5
					$\leq E = 2.0$

[a]Geometric mean $= \dfrac{\leq E}{f} = \dfrac{2.0}{5} = 0.4$

Source: Ref. 39.

the product sample and the water control sample are compared.
If the product sample mean is within twofold of the control mean
sample, the drug product is judged not to inhibit or enhance the
LAL-endotoxin reaction. For example, if the product sample
showed a geometric mean of 0.4 EU/ml and the water control
mean was 0.2 EU/ml, the LAL test is valid for that product.

If endotoxin is detectable in the untreated specimens under the
conditions of the test, the product is unsuitable for the inhibition/
enhancement test. Either endotoxin must be removed by ultrafiltration or further dilution can be made as long as the MVD is
not exceeded and the inhibition/enhancement test repeated. If
the drug product is found to cause inhibition or enhancement of
the LAL test, the following courses of action can be taken (42):

1. If the drug product is amenable to rabbit testing, then the
    rabbit test will still be the appropriate pyrogen test for
    that drug.

2. If the interfering substances can be neutralized without affecting the sensitivity of the test or if the LAL test is more sensitive than the rabbit pyrogen test, then the LAL test can still be used.
3. For those drugs not amenable to rabbit pyrogen testing the manufacturer should demonstrate that the LAL test can detect the endotoxin limit established for the particular drug. If the limit cannot be met, the smallest quantity of endotoxin that can be detected must be determined.

There are various miscellaneous requirements in the procedures for validating the LAL test:

1. Use positive and negative controls in all tests.
2. Use the highest and lowest drug concentrations for drug products marketed in three or more concentrations.
3. Use three lots of each drug concentration for the validation tests.
4. If the lysate manufacturer is changed, validation test must be repeated on at least one unit of product.
5. The LAL reagent should have a sensitivity of at least 0.25 EU/ml.
6. The endotoxin control must always be referenced to the RSE.
7. Any change in the product formulation, manufacturing process, source of formulation ingredients, or lot of lysate necessitates a re-validation of the LAL test for the product.

Devices

A sensitivity of at least 0.1 mg/ml of *E. coli* 055:B5 endotoxin or its equivalent (e.g., RSE can be used if it correlates to 055:B5) must be demonstrated in the testing laboratory using an FDA-licensed LAL reagent. If the testing laboratory will also be using the rabbit pyrogen test for re-testing purposes, the endotoxin sensitivity in the rabbit colony must be ≤ 0.1 ng/ml (i.e., 0.1 ng/ml in 10 ml/kg dose will produce a pyrogenic reaction in rabbits). The methods used for determining sensitivity in devices are essentially the same as those used for drugs and biologics.

The possibility of a device inhibiting or enhancing the LAL-endotoxin reaction is determined by extraction testing of each of three device production lots. The extract solution must be pyrogen-free water or saline to which known amounts of standard endotoxin, bracketing the sensitivity of the lysate, have been added. Depending on the type of device, extracts may be obtained by flushing, immersing, or disassembling, then immersing the device with the endotoxin-spiked solution. The LAL test results of the extract should not be different than the results of testing standard solutions containing endotoxin that have not been exposed to the device.

Manual LAL Test Procedure

Four or more replicate samples at each level of the dilution series for the test samples are used in most cases. The pH of the reaction mixture must be between 6.0 and 7.5 unless specified differently in the particular monograph. The pH may be adjusted by addition of sterile, endotoxin-free 0.1 N sodium hydroxide or 0.1 N hydrochloric acid or suitable buffers.

Test tubes, usually of the dimensions 10 by 75 mm, are filled with an aliquot, usually 0.1 ml, of reconstituted LAL reagent, and the same aliquot volume of the test sample. In other test tubes, equal volumes of LAL reagent and endotoxin standard are combined. Positive controls (LAL reagent sample containing a known concentration of endotoxin) and negative controls (LAL reagent + equal volume of sterile, pyrogen-free solvent) are run simultaneously with the test samples and endotoxin standards.

When the equal volumes are combined, the test tube is swirled gently. The tube is placed in a constant temperature water bath with temperature controlled at 37 ± 1°C. Incubation times ideally last 60 ± 2 minutes. While incubating, the test tubes must never be disturbed for fear of irreversibly disengaging the gel clot if it has formed. Careful removal of the incubated test tubes for gel clot analysis is extremely important.

The use of microscope slides containing petrolatum wells has been advocated for conducting the LAL test when lower reagent consumption is desired (43). One slide can accommodate 12 samples using microliter volumes (0.1 μl). A dye solution (0.1% toluidine blue in ethanol) is placed in each well to aid in interpreting the results. A positive LAL test generates a blue "star" in the droplet while a negative LAL test gives a homogenous blue solution.

The degree of gel formation can be determined by either direct visual observation or instrumental analysis. Visual observation starts by carefully removing the test tube from the incubator, then carefully inverting (by 180 degrees) the test tube and visually checking for the appearance of a firm gel. A positive reaction is characterized by the formation of a firm gel that does not break or lose its integrity during and at the completion of the inversion process. A negative result is characterized by the absence of a gel or by formation of a viscous gel that does not maintain its integrity during the inversion process. Examples of a positive and a negative LAL test result are seen in Figure 2.11.

Instrumental Tests

Direct visual observation of the gel endpoint relies on the subjective interpretation of the observer and, unless twofold serial dilutions are performed, provides only a qualitative (yes or no) measurement of the endotoxin present in the sample. Analysis of the gel endpoint by instrumental methods offers several advantages, including single-tube quantitation and objectivity. Additionally, instrumental methods can be automated, resulting in increased speed, efficiency, and adaptation to computer control.

Two basic instrumental methods are available for LAL testing. One method is based on turbidimetric measurement of gel formation (e.g., Abbott's MS-2, Millipore's Pyrostat), while the other method is based on colorimetrically measuring a chromophoric substance produced during the LAL-endotoxin reaction (e.g., Mallinckrodt and Whittaker M.A. Bioproducts).

The Abbott MS-2 Microbiology System was designed originally for automated antibiotic susceptibility testing of clinical samples. The system was first described by Jorgensen and Alexander (44) and later by Novitsky et al. (45). A general procedure is outlined below:

1. LAL is mixed with the test sample in a 1:4 ratio, e.g., 100 µl LAL + 400 µl test, in a polystyrene research cuvette.
2. Up to 88 samples can be incubated per module. Incubation occurs at 35°C for 60 minutes.
3. The mixture of each cuvette following incubation is examined for turbidity (light transmission) by recording the optical density (OD) at 670 nm on the MS-2 spectrophotometer. The samples are examined at either one- or five-minute intervals.
4. The OD values are recorded on a cassette tape and/or paper and can be displayed graphically as OD vs. time on a cathode ray tube or transferred to paper with a hard copy printer. An example of a plot of OD at 670 nm vs. time using standard endotoxin samples is shown in Figure 2.12 (45).

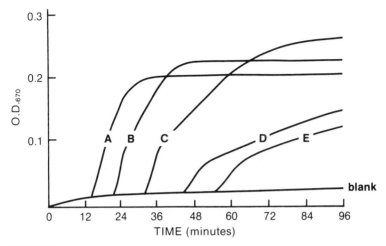

FIGURE 2.12 Turbidimetric response of LAL with control standard endotoxin diluted in sterile water for irrigation. A, 100 pg
endotoxin/nl; B, 25 pg/nl; C, 6.3 pg/nl; D, 1.6 pg/nl; E, 0.4
pg/nl. (From Ref. 45.)

Turbidimetric optical density has been shown to be directly proportional to *E. coli* endotoxin concentration on a log-log plot. For
example, Figure 2.13 shows such a relationship. Standard curves
usually are linear only within a relatively small concentration
range, e.g., 0.01−0.1 ng/ml (0.1−1.0 EU/ml). The establishment of standrd curves for instrumental analyses of the LAL-
endotoxin reaction can be difficult. The availability of standard
endotoxin has improved the reproducibility of standard curve
determinations.

A practical example of the use of the Abbott MS-2 automated
LAL test system in the detection of bacteriuria was published by
Jorgensen and Alexander (46). The use of turbidimetry in
automated LAL testing provided a way of successfully analyzing
endotoxin in blood (47). Automated microliter testing overcomes
the inhibitory factors in blood which mask the gelatin reaction
using conventional LAL test methodology.

A newer type of automated LAL test system is based on the
measurement of color intensity of the LAL gel endpoint. This
system is called the Chromogenic LAL assay system (Figure 2.14).
Test sample is mixed with LAL reagent and incubated at 37°C for
a period of time (usually 10 minutes). A substrate solution containing a color-producing substance is then mixed with the LAL

QUANTITATION

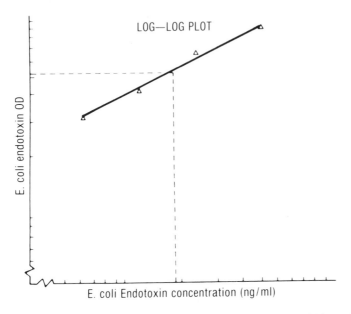

FIGURE 2.13   Log-log relationship between turbidimetric optical density and endotoxin concentration. (Courtesy of the Millipore Corporation, Bedford, Massachusetts.)

test sample and incubated at 37°C for an additional three minutes. The reaction is stopped with 50% acetic acid. The color absorbancy of the sample mixture is determined spectrophotometrically at 405 nm. The more intense the color, the greater the absorbance value measured. Endotoxin concentration can then be determined from a standard plot of absorbance vs. endotoxin concentration in ng/ml or EU/ml.

The chemical composition of the substrate is a peptide chain linked to p-nitroaniline (pNA) (48). The endotoxin catalyzes the activation of a proenzyme in the LAL as discussed on pages 100—101. The activated enzyme, in turn, catalyzes the splitting of pNA from the colorless substrate. In Figure 2.10 pNA replaces coagulogen as the substance cleaved by the proenzyme. It is pNA that is measured spectrophotometrically. Absorbance at 405 nm and endotoxin concentration are linearly related between 0.01 and 0.1 ng/ml.

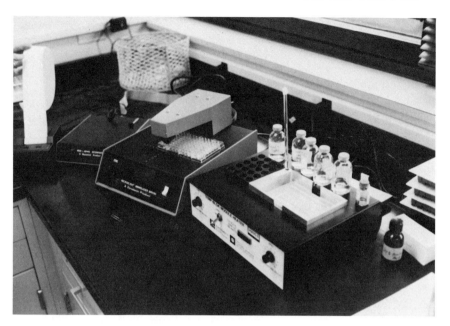

FIGURE 2.14   Chromogenic LAL assay system. (Courtesy of
Whittaker M.A. Bioproducts, Walkersville, Maryland.)

For laboratories responsible for conducting multiple LAL tests,
automation practically becomes a necessity. Automation employs
all the advantages of instrumental analyses, including greater
precision and sensitivity. The major disadvantages of automated
LAL testing systems are their cost and complexity. Cooper (49)
recommended that each laboratory carefully consider its present
and long-term needs as well as being firmly grounded in the
fundamentals of the LAL test before changing from manual to
automated LAL test systems.

Appendix V at the end of this book presents a comparison of
published LAL methodology courtesy of a review article by
Novitsky (50).

The LAL test requirements for lack of pyrogenicity or critical
endotoxin concentration will be met if there is no formation of a
firm gel at the level of endotoxin specified in the individual monograph. For instances where instrumental analyses have been
done, the sample will pass the LAL test if not more than the
maximum permissible amount of endotoxin specified in the individual

monograph is present in the sample. Additionally, the confidence limits of the assay must not exceed the limits previously specified for the instrumental analysis.

Endotoxin Limits in Parenteral Articles

The first FDA draft guideline for LAL testing of drugs (51) proposed an endotoxin limit for all parenterals of 0.25 EU/ml. This limit was vehemently opposed by the parenteral drug industry because the limit was arbitrary, based on concentration rather than endotoxin quantity per dose, and did not permit sufficient dilution of small-volume parenterals known to inhibit the LAL test reaction.

The Parenteral Drug Association proposed an alternative endotoxin limit based on rabbit or human dose (52) that FDA accepted and became part of the new FDA draft guideline for end product testing published in March, 1983 (42). The new endotoxin limit is

$$\frac{K}{M} = \frac{\text{Threshold Pyrogen Dose (TPD)}}{\text{Maximum rabbit or human dose}}$$

where the TPD has been defined as 5 EU/kg, the lower 95% confidence limit of the average dose found to produce a pyrogenic response in rabbits (53). For drugs administered intrathecally, where pyrogenic contamination can be much more dangerous (see page 125), the TPD is 0.2 EU/kg.

The maximum rabbit or human dose is that dose administered per kg of body weight of rabbit or man in a single hour period, whichever is larger. For example, if a drug of a concentration of 1 mg/ml has a maximum human loading of 25 mg/kg while the rabbit pyrogen test dose is 10 mg/kg, the maximum dose used in the denominator of the endotoxin limit equation would be the human dose of of 25 mg. On the other hand, were the above human dose only 2.5 mg/kg, then the rabbit dose of 10 mg would be the larger of the two doses. The endotoxin limit for the two examples would be:

$$EU = \frac{5 \text{ EU/kg}}{25 \text{ mg/kg}} = 0.2 \text{ EU/mg}$$

$$EU = \frac{5 \text{ EU/kg}}{10 \text{ mg/kg}} = 0.5 \text{ EU/mg}$$

For devices, the endotoxin limit is 0.1 ng per milliliter of extract solution.

Four classes of drugs are exempted from the endotoxin limit defined by K/M:

1. Compendial drugs for which other endotoxin limits have been established
2. Drugs covered by new drug applications, antibiotic Form 5 and Form 6 applications, new animal drug applications, and biological product license where different limits have been approved by the Agency
3. Investigational drugs or biologics for which an IND or INAD exemption has been filed and approved
4. Drugs or biologics that cannot be tested by the LAL method

Sensitivity of LAL

LAL sensitivity is defined as the lowest concentration of a purified endotoxin that will produce a firm gel, which will remain intact when inverted carefully after one hour of incubation at 37°C. (LAL sensitivity is also expressed as how many times its sensitivity is greater than the rabbit test.) In general, it seems to be well established that the LAL test is sensitive to picogram quantities of endotoxin and that LAL is from 5 to 50 times more sensitive than the rabbit to the presence of endotoxin, depending on the type of comparative study conducted.

Earlier studies by Cooper et al. (32) demonstrated that the LAL test was at least five times more sensitive to purified endotoxin than was the rabbit test. This was later confirmed by Elin and Wolff (54). Improvements in LAL production and formulation methodology increased the sensitivity of LAL 10 to 50 times greater than the rabbit test (40,55). These numbers were based on a gel time of one hour and a rabbit test dose of 1 ml/kg.

Ronneberger (56) found that the LAL test gave similar results or was 10 times more sensitive than the rabbit test using lipopoly-saccharides from different gram negative bacteria (see Table 2.9). In more than 300 samples of drugs, plasma proteins, and other antigens, the LAL test and rabbit test gave similar results, although the lower sensitivity of the rabbit test had to be compensated for by injection of a higher volume of test sample.

Marcus and Nelson (30) have stated that the rabbit pyrogen assay will detect 1 to 10 ng of enterobacterial endotoxin while the LAL test will detect 0.01 to 0.1 ng endotoxin per ml solution.

TABLE 2.9 LAL Specificity and Sensitivity for the Detection of
Lipopolysaccharides

LPS source	Minimum dose for positive rabbit response[a]	Minimum conc. for positive LAL reaction[b]
Salmonella typhi Type 58	1 ng	0.1 ng/0.1 ml
Salmonella abort. equi	10 ng	10 pg/0.1 ml
Lipid A of Salmonella abort. equi	100 pg	10 pg/0.1 ml
Salmonella minnesot.	10 pg	1 pg/0.1 ml
E. coli	10 ng	0.1 ng/0.1 ml
Klebsiella pneumoniae	1 ng	2 ng no reaction

[a]Three rabbits used.
[b]LAL source: Pyrogent (Mallinckrodt).
Source: From Ref. 56.

Table 2.10 Sensitivity of the Rabbit Pyrogen Test and of the
Limulus Test in the Detection of E. coli Endotoxin

ng/ml	Rabbit pyrogen test[a]	Limulus test
500	Pyrogenic	Positive
50	Pyrogenic	Positive
5	Non-pyrogenic	Positive
0.5	Non-pyrogenic	Positive
0.05	–	Negative
0.005	–	Negative

[a]Dose: 1 ml endotoxin solution/kg body weight.
Source: From Ref. 57.

The ability of LAL to detect *E. coli* endotoxin in pyrogen-free distilled water was found to be 100 times more sensitive than the rabbit test (see Table 2.10) (57).

Lysate sensitivity will vary according to commercial source of the lysate, as is the case with endotoxin sensitivity. Wachtel and Tsuji (58) tested six commercial lysate preparations against *E. coli* endotoxin. Sensitivity ranged from 0.3 to 0.003 ng/ml. Similar results were found with endotoxins extracted from *Salmonella typhosa*, *Serratia marcescens*, and *Shigella flexneri*. *Pseudomonas* sensitivity ranged from 10 ng/ml to as high as 500 ng/ml.

Twohy et al. (59) compared lysates from five LAL manufacturers (Associates of Cape Cod, Difco, Haemachem, M. A. Bioproducts, and Mallinckrodt). Using the gel-clot method with nine different drug products and EC-5 endotoxin standard, these investigators found that endpoints varied among the LAL reagents from the different manufacturers. Lot-to-lot variability with LAL reagents from two manufacturers was observed as well as the ability of some LAL reagents to change the pH of the drug product. These data support the fact that some LAL reagents are better suited for some drug products than for other products and that the LAL test must be revalidated for every drug product when LAL manufacturers and/or LAL lots are changed.

Sensitivity of LAL for endotoxin depends greatly on the vehicle in which the endotoxin is contained. For example, LAL can detect only 5 to 10 mcg/ml endotoxin in plasma whereas 0.05 mcg/ml endotoxin was detectable in cerebrospinal fluid (60). The failure of LAL to detect known levels of endotoxin in human serum albumin and other protein solutions is well known (39). Many drug products inhibit the LAL test and severely retard its sensitivity. These inhibitions and limitations of the LAL test will be discussed in the section "Limitations of the LAL Test."

LAL Test Specificity

Whereas sensitivity is the ability of a test to give positive reactions in the presence of the material tested, specificity is the ability of a test to give positive reactions with only the material tested (30). The sensitivity of LAL toward endotoxin is undisputed. However, its specificity in reacting solely with endotoxin is its most controversial characteristic.

In 1973 Elin and Wolff (54) first reported the possible lack of specificity of the LAL test for bacterial endotoxin. Substances found to cause lysate gelatin included thrombin, thromboplastin, ribonucleases, and polynucleotides such as polyriboadenylic acid

and polyribouridylic acid. Wildfeuer et al. (61) found that pep-
tidoglycans isolated from various gram positive bacteria caused
lysate gelatin. Positive reactions have been found between LAL
and streptococcal exotoxins (62), synthetic dextrans (63), lipoteichoic acids (64), and the dithiols, dithiothreitol and dithio-
erythritol (65).

Person and Weary (66) addressed these false positive reactions
caused by nonendotoxin substances. They concluded that such
substances need not concern parenteral drug manufacturers because of one or more of the following reasons: (a) Many of the
substances (including all of the synthetic substances) would not
be found in a parenteral product. (b) The substance may be
present, but not in sufficient concentrations to produce gelation
in lysate or fever in rabbits. (c) The substance is a highly purified preparation that could not occur in production. (d) Results
have not been confirmed by other researchers. (e) Because a
negative LAL test result demonstrates the unequivocal absence
of endotoxin, concern over false positives becomes a moot point
with proper positive and negative controls. Concerns over false
negatives can be eliminated by the same validation process. For
example, the clotting enzyme in LAL, coagulogen, is similar bio-
chemically to trypsin. Trypsin, in turn, can initiate the gelation
reaction (33). To be certain that a positive LAL test is due unequivocally to endotoxin contamination, adequate controls are
used to demonstrate that substances like trypsin are not the cause
of the gelation observed.

Advantages of the LAL Test Compared to the USP Rabbit Test

Proponents of the LAL test claim that the test offers at least
seven advantages over the use of the USP rabbit test for detecting
pyrogens in parenteral injectable products and medical devices
(24):

1. Greater sensitivity
2. Greater reliability
3. Better specificity
4. Less variation
5. Wider application
6. Use as a problem-solving tool
7. Less expensive

The majority of these advantages are a direct result of the remarkable simplicity of the LAL test. Being an in vitro test requiring a minimal number of items to complete the test, LAL offers rapidity and reliability unmatched by an in vivo system.

Control of technique, handling, and external environmental factors are achieved much more easily with the LAL test. This, in turn, leads to minimized chances of error and variation in the testing results. The ease and adaptability of the LAL test allow it to be used in many different situations for which application of the rabbit test would be impractical or impossible. In fact, the need for a rapid, simple, and sensitive technique for pyrogen testing of extemporaneously prepared radiopharmaceutical preparations led to some of the earliest applied research involving the LAL test in hospital pharmacy quality control. Other applications of the LAL test, rendered possible because of its unique advantages compared to the rabbit test, include pyrogen testing of in-process water for injection, bacterial and viral vaccines, antineoplastic agents, drugs designed for intrathecal injection, and validation of dry heat depyrogenation cycles. These applications will be elaborated in the section "LAL Test Applications."

The LAL test has become an acceptable substitute for the rabbit test in the in-process pyrogen control of plasma fractions (67). Four advantages given for substituting the LAL test in place of the rabbit test were: (a) employing an in vitro test, when available, rather than an animal test; (b) results are available within 90 minutes after beginning the test procedure; (c) tests can be conducted with LAL when using the rabbit test would be senseless because of the time factor; (d) the LAL test is simple and inexpensive.

Fumarola and Jirillo (68) stated that according to some 140 papers reported in the literature dealing with the LAL test, as well as their own experience, the test is an acceptable, specific, rapid, and sensitive method for endotoxin assay of parenteral drugs and biological products, and for in-process testing of parenteral solutions.

Researchers at Travenol Laboratories have published many articles providing data to support the superiority of the LAL test over the rabbit test for pyrogen testing of large-volume parenterals (LVPs) (24, 69—71). Their arguments were summarized by Mascoli and Weary (24):

1. Pyrogens important in LVP products and devices are endotoxin in nature.

2. After tens of thousands of tests, an unexplained negative LAL test result-positive rabbit test result was never recorded.
3. Some endotoxin pyrogens detected by LAL were not detected by rabbit tests.
4. In some cases, the rabbit test results only failed initially to detect pyrogens that were sometimes confirmed later by rabbit tests but were always confirmed by initial LAL tests.

In a poll taken by this author of quality control representatives from 10 pharmaceutical manufacturers of parenteral products and devices, 7 of 10 responded that they preferred the LAL test over the rabbit test. The advantages of the LAL test as reasons given for their preference were (in order of importance):

1. Greater sensitivity
2. Less variation
3. Quantitative results
4. Less time-consuming
5. Less expensive
6. An easier test

Limitations of the LAL Test

Unquestionably, the LAL test fills the need for a simple, sensitive, accurate, and inexpensive method for detecting bacterial endotoxin. It certainly offers itself as an excellent alternative or supplemental method to the official USP rabbit test for pyrogen. However, it is not without limitations or problems.

The greatest limitation of the LAL test is the problem of interference of the lysate-endotoxin interaction that is caused by a variety of drugs and other substances (72–75). Seven of the 10 quality control representatives from the parenteral industry polled by the author identified inhibition of the lysate-endotoxin interaction as the number one factor limiting the applicability of the LAL test. As discussed on page 101, the LAL gelation reaction is mediated by a clotting enzyme that is heat labile, pH sensitive, and chemically related to trypsin (76–77). Inhibition is caused by any material known to denature protein or to inhibit enzyme action. A representative listing of drugs and other substances known to modify or inhibit the lysate-endotoxin interaction is given in Table 2.11. Inhibition by many drug components can be over-

TABLE 2.11   Examples of Small Volume Parenterals Reported to Markedly Inhibit the LAL Test

Inhibition overcome by more than one twofold dilution	Inhibition at maximum valid dilution
Aminophylline injection	Carbazochrome salicylate
Ascorbic acid and vitamin B complex injection	Cyclizine lactate
Chorionic gonadotropin	Diatrizoate meglumine and diatrizoate sodium
Clindamycin phosphate	Edetate disodium injection
Cyanocobalamin injection	Fluorescein sodium
Dicyclomine hydrochloride	Liver injection
Diphenydramine hydrochloride	Meperidine hydrochloride and promethazine hydrochloride
Dyphylline injection	Oxacillin sodium
Ephedrine hydrochloride	Pentamidine isethionate
Fluorouracil	Peptonized iron large volume parenteral
Lidocaine hydrochloride	Sulfisoxazole
Lidocaine hydrochloride and epinephrine	Sulfobromophthalein sodium
Meperidine hydrochloride injection	Vancomycin hydrochloride
Mepivacaine hydrochloride and levonordefrin	
Multi-vitamin injection	
Promethazine hydrochloride	
Scopolamine hydrobromide	
Tetracaine hydrochloride	
Thiamine hydrochloride	

Source: C. W. Twohy, A. P. Duran, and T. E. Munson, *J. Parenteral Sci. Tech.*, *38*, 190−201, (1984).

come by dilution or pH adjustment. Of course, dilution reduces the concentration of the endotoxin and places greater demand on the sensitivity of the LAL reagent to detect diluted amounts of endotoxin.

Tests for inhibition or activation basically involve the use of positive controls. Product samples are "spiked" with known endotoxin levels, preferably the same levels used in standards prepared for sensitivity determinations. The endpoint of detection for the product sample should be no different from the endpoint for the standard series. In other words, if the lowest standard detectable level of endotoxin is 0.025 ng/ml, this level must also be detectable by the same lot of LAL reagent in the product sample. If inhibition is found to occur, serial dilutions of the product sample are made until the appropriate dilution is found that no longer modifies the gelation reaction.

Other concerns or limitations of the LAL test are:

1. LAL is dependable only for the detection of pyrogen originating from gram negative bacteria.
2. Being an in vitro test, the LAL test cannot measure the fever-producing potential of endotoxin present in the sample.
3. The sensitivity of LAL varies appreciably with endotoxins from various microbial sources.
4. It is difficult to compare the sensitivity of the LAL test and the rabbit test because the rabbit assay is dose dependent while the LAL test is concentration dependent.
5. Gel formation can be difficult to interpret and can be broken upon the slightest vibration.
6. The LAL test is too sensitive in that it can detect endotoxin at levels below those required for producing fever in mammals. Yet the FDA may enforce a level of sensitivity for the LAL test much greater than that for the rabbit test. In other words, a product that will consistently pass the USP pyrogen test may not pass the LAL test. Does this mean that the product is pyrogenic and harmful to man?
7. Extensive studies are required to validate the LAL test as the final product pyrogen test.

LAL Test Applications

From a modest beginning of detecting endotoxin in blood, LAL test application has expanded into a variety of laboratory and clinical situations. New or improved usage of the LAL test appears in the literature on a monthly basis. As the methodology becomes more standardized, as reference standards become more accepted, and as automatic instrumental analysis becomes further developed, LAL testing for endotoxin in the parenteral field will become standard practice just as other quality control methods have.

At this time the LAL test has been used as an indicator of endotoxin contamination in at least six different areas:

1. Pharmaceuticals
2. Biologicals
3. Devices
4. Disease states
5. Food
6. Validation of depyrogenation cycles

The literature is massive with regard to LAL test applications in most of these areas. Not all published reports will be discussed, but those with significant impact will be described in the following subsections. Reference 78 is a good source of plentiful articles dealing with applications of the LAL test.

Pharmaceuticals

While LAL has found considerable application in processing and final product quality control procedures of parenteral pharmaceuticals, the FDA Bureau of Drugs only recently has approved the test as a final products release test for pyrogens. For years the LAL test has been used in many situations to support product release in the industry and to qualify certain hospital-prepared products.

Radiopharmaceuticals represent a special class of parenteral medications for which the LAL test offers unique advantages in the detection of pyrogen contamination. Many radiopharmaceuticals are prepared extemporaneously, such as technetium 99m (99mTc), which has a biological half-life of only six to seven hours. The LAL test, because of its short time for testing, low volume requirements, and low cost, obviously is the preferred method for pyrogen detection in radiopharmaceuticals. DeMurphy and Aneiros (79) used a micro LAL test method for pyrogen detection in 204 radiopharmaceuticals including pertechnetate, sulfur colloid, pyrophosphates, pyridoxylidenglutamate, human serum albumin, and human albumin macroaggregates. They concluded that the test proved to be economic, easy, rapid, sensitive, and reliable. The test was incorporated into the routine quality control program not only for radiopharmaceuticals, but also for all parenteral fluids and solutions used in kit preparation within their nuclear medicine department.

Rhodes and Croft (80) listed six reasons why the LAL test is preferred over the rabbit test for pyrogen testing of radiopharmaceuticals and reagent kits:

1. It is more sensitive.
2. It is faster.

3. It requires smaller amounts of test material.
4. Both positive and negative controls can be performed along with each test.
5. It does not generate radioactive rabbits so it is preferred from a radiologic safety point of view.
6. It is less expensive and easier to store.

Antineoplastic agents are another class of parenteral medications for which the LAL test provides marked advantages over the USP rabbit test. Endotoxin is an expected contaminant of the enzyme L-asparaginase (33) because it is obtained from cultures of *E. coli* ATCC 9637. However, the USP pyrogen test cannot be used to detect endotoxin in this preparation because the rabbit is one of the species extremely susceptible to the toxic effect of the enzyme (81). L-asparaginase and bleomycin contain as much as 50 ng/ml endotoxin (82). It is suspected that this contaminant is the cause of the adverse effects seen in patients following administration of these agents. The LAL test sensitivity characteristics aid in evaluating the techniques applied to reduce or eliminate the endotoxin level in these agents.

The LAL test has been used to detect the presence of bacterial endotoxin in 12 chemotherapeutic agents currently in use clinically (83). Relative concentrations of endotoxin ranging from 0.1 to 63 ng/ml were detected in individual lots of the following drugs: L-asparaginase, 5-azacytidine, bleomycin, DTIC, antinomycin D, adriamycin, and vinblastine. On the other hand, all lots of the following antineoplastic agents contained ⩽0.1 ng/ml endotoxin: cytosine arabinoside, cyclophosphamide, daunorubicin, vincristine, and streptozotocin. The authors concluded that the LAL test is a rapid and specific method for detection of small amounts of bacterial endotoxin contaminating parenteral preparations of antitumor agents.

Antibiotics are known to inhibit the LAL test at the product concentrations used in human or animal dosages. In most cases, however, adequate dilution of most of these products above the minimum valid concentration (MVC) will provide non-inhibitory for successful application of the LAL test. Case et al. (84) tested 28 antibiotics with the LAL assay to determine their non-inhibitory concentrations (NICs). Most of the antibiotics tested could be diluted to NICs above the MVCs. Five antibiotic products presented problems. Cefamandole nafate and neomycin sulfate had NICs very close to their MVCs (1.6:0.8 mg/ml and 0.2:0.16 mg/ml, respectively). Polymyxin B and colistimethate contained too much endotoxin to permit determination of their NICs. The NIC of tetracycline hydrochloride was dependent on the initial concentration of the antibiotic. If the initial concentration of tetracycline was 5 mg/ml, dilution to 0.16 mg/ml produced a non-inhibitory concentration that was less than the MVC for tetracycline. However, a concentration of 0.5 mg/ml, when diluted, produced a NIC about the same as the MVC. The reason for this difference probably was the amount of NaOH required to adjust the pH of this very acidic antibiotic solution (pH = 2.8). The greater amount of base required to increase pH of the 5.0 mg/ml product probably caused too high a sodium ion concentration for the LAL test to overcome.

Other pharmaceutical preparations for which the LAL test holds promise as a final product release test for pyrogens include large-volume parenterals (85), intravenous fat emulsions (86), iron dextran (87), and most of the drug products listed in Table 2.11. Despite the need for dilution to eliminate the inhibitory effects of many small-volume parenteral drug products, the LAL test is claimed to be at least equal to or more sensitive than the USP pyrogen test (88, 89).

Pharmaceuticals administered by the intrathecal route represent a drug class most urgently in need of the LAL test for endotoxin detection (40). Such pharmaceuticals include (a) dyes such as methylene blue and fluorescein for detecting cerebrospinal fluid (CSF) leakage, (b) contrast media for visualization of CSF pathways, (c) cancer chemotherapeutic agents such as methotrexate for treatment of leukemic meningitis, (d) antibiotics such as gentamicin for septic meningitis, and (e) radiopharmaceuticals for radionuclide cisternography, a procedure wherein a small volume of radiotracer is administered intrathecally to study CSF dynamics by means of nuclear imaging devices. Endotoxin has been shown to be extremely more toxic following intrathecal injection compared to intravenous injection. For example, Bennett and co-workers (90) demonstrated in animals that instillation of endotoxin into intrathecal spaces was at least 1000 times more potent in producing a febrile response than the intravenous route.

The USP rabbit pyrogen test for intrathecal drugs has been shown to be insufficiently sensitive to serve as a screening test for endotoxin contamination of these drugs (40). Thus, the LAL test should replace or at least supplement the USP pyrogen test for drugs intended to be administered into CSF.

Biologics

The FDA's Bureau of Biologics (BoB) in 1977 published conditions under which the LAL test can be applied as the end-product pyrogen test for biologics (see page 99). The main requirement involves validating that the LAL test and rabbit test are at least equivalent for each product undergoing pyrogen testing.

The LAL test has been used both for end-product testing and for solving problems during the manufacturing of blood products and plasma fractions. Expediency, sensitivity, and quantitation of endotoxin levels are three advantages of using the LAL test rather than the rabbit test. A comparison of the two pyrogen tests as they are applied to various biological substances was reported by Ronneberger (56), and an example of his data is given in Table 2.12.

LAL assays have been demonstrated as satisfactory for three primary biological substances: human serum albumin (66, 91), plasma fractions (56, 67, 92), and vaccines (93). However, human serum in toto inhibits the LAL gelation reaction with spiked endotoxin unless modifications in the test procedure are incorporated. Human serum contains a single protein (designated LPS-1) that inactivates LPS and inhibits the gelation reaction (94). Other inhibitors are present in serum such as two alpha-globulins (95) and a serum globulin esterase (96). Another variable is that the levels of substances inhibiting endotoxin probably vary not only from person to person, but also in a patent during various stages of illness associated with gram negative infections (97).

Three methods have been reported that are capable of removing these serum inhibitors. They include extracting the serum with chloroform (98), adjusting the plasma pH (99), and combining the application of heat and serum dilution to overcome the inhibiting capacity of the inhibitors (100).

Baek (101) has reported an immunoelectrophoretic assay that greatly improves the sensitivity of LAL for lipopolysaccharide detection in various biological fluids including plasma. The assay method is based on the preparation of a monospecific antibody against coagulogen, the clottable protein formed in the LAL-endotoxin reaction (see the section "LAL Reaction Mechanism"). As coagulogen splits into coagulin and C-peptide, the antigenicity of the cleaved coagulogen is lost, and this is expressed by a diminished migration of the protein on the rocket immunoelectrophoresis (RIE) plate. The method increased lipopolysaccharide detectability in plasma by 1000 times, i.e., from 1 ng LPS/ml of plasma by visual LAL testing to 1 pg LPS/ml plasma using RIE.

Devices

In a *Federal Register* notice on November 4, 1977 (42FR:57749), the LAL test was approved by the Bureau of Medical Devices of

TABLE 2.12 Comparison of LAL and Rabbit Tests on Various Materials

Material	No. of samples	Dose rabbit ml/kg I.V.	Rabbit[a] +	Rabbit[a] −	LAL[b] dose 0.1 ml +	LAL[b] dose 0.1 ml −	Rabbit − LAL +
Haemaccel plasma substitute	35	10	2	33	2	33	0
Physiologic saline	21	10	2	19	2	19	0
Aqua dest.	25	10	3	22	3	22	0
Albumin human	65	3	21	44	31	34	10
Gammaglobulin	31	1	8	23	16	15	8
F(ab)$_2$-fragment	27	3	8	19	12	15	4
Plasma protein solution	18	3	44	14	9	9	5
Fibrinogen	6	1.5	1	5	3	3	2
Factor XIII	10	1	2	8	2	8	0
Proteinase inhibitor							
ANTAGOSAN	9	2	1	8	1	8	0
Interferon	6	1	4	2	5	1	1
Streptokinase	35	1	3	32	5	30	2

TABLE 2.12 (Continued)

Material	No. of samples	Dose rabbit ml/kg I.V.	Rabbit[a]		LAL[b] dose 0.1 ml		Rabbit − LAL +
			+	−	+	−	
Neuraminidase	12	1	4	8	6	6	2
Vaccines div.	45	0.5 - 10	24	21	26	21	2
	345	0.5 - 10	87	248	123	222	36
Plasma human treated chloroform	28	1	18	10	5	23	

[a]Rabbit + = Plasma 13.
  LAL − = Plasma 13.
[b]LAL: Pyrogent.
Other samples: 4.
Source: Ref. 56.

the FDA (now the National Center for Devices and Radiological Health, NCDRH) as a suitable test to replace the USP pyrogen test for final release of medical devices. As with the biologics, the manufacturer may use the LAL test as a final release test for devices only after meeting four conditions:

1. Demonstrate the equivalence of the LAL test and rabbit test for each device.
2. Document the proficiency in applying the LAL test.
3. Describe LAL test methodology in detail.
4. Determine acceptance limits for the applicable device products.

NCDRH recently eliminated the requirement for prior FDA approval to use the LAL test as an end-product test for devices when it is used according to current FDA guidelines. However, all validation data required prior to releasing devices labeled nonpyrogenic based on the LAL test must be kept on file at the manufacturing site and be available for FDA inspection (102). If a manufacturer plans to use LAL test procedures that differ significantly from FDA guidelines, then the manufacturer must submit either a 510(k) or a premarket approval supplement.

Hundreds of device manufacturers in the United States as well as in foreign countries have taken advantage of the opportunity to replace the rabbit test with the LAL test. The major barrier that must be solved for a device manufacturer to receive regulatory approval to use the LAL test involves the validation of the equivalency of the two pyrogen test methods.

Representatives of HIMA took the initiative to propose guidelines (103) and conduct studies (104) to help the medical device manufacturer successfully design and carry out procedures for LAL pyrogen testing. The guidelines suggested are summarized in Figure 2.15. The collaborative study conducted under HIMA auspices evaluated the pyrogenecity of *E. coli* 055:B5 from Difco Laboratories (Detroit). Using 12 rabbit colonies provided by device manufacturers, contract testing laboratories, and the FDA, the average pyrogenic dose of *E. coli* 055:B5 endotoxin was found to be 0.157 ng/ml (1.57 ng/kg for 10 ml/kg injected dose). The lower 95% confidence level was 0.1 ng/ml, meaning that if eight rabbits were administered this concentration of endotoxin, four rabbits would fail the pyrogen test at this dose. Therefore, any device manufacturer wishing to use the LAL test must validate the ability of their test procedure to detect Difco *E. coli* 055:B5 endotoxin at levels at least equivalent to 0.1 ng/ml (1.0 ng/kg dose).

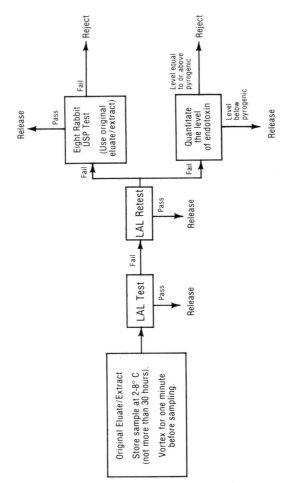

FIGURE 2.15 Schematic flow chart of the guidelines proposed by HIMA for LAL pyrogen testing of medical devices. (From M. Weary and F. Pearson, Pyrogen testing with Limulus amebocyte lysate, *Med. Device Diag.*, Nov. 1980. Copyright 1980, Cannon Communications, Inc.)

NCDRH requires the following sampling guidelines to be used for different device lot sites:

Two devices for lots of less than 30
Three devices for lots of 30—100
3% of lots above 100 up to a maximum of 10 devices per lot

The recommended volume of non-pyrogenic rinsing fluid per device is 40 ml. If 10 devices are rinsed, then the total rinsing extract pooled is 400 ml. If a rinse volume greater than 40 ml per device is required, a more sensitive LAL endpoint should be used.

Disease States

Because endotoxins are associated with gram negative bacteria, diseases caused by these bacteria conceivably can be diagnosed by the LAL test. A partial list of gram negative bacteria is given in Table 2.13 along with diseases associated with these organisms.

Endotoxemia is a low-grade infection of the intestinal tract caused by bacterial endotoxins. Endotoxemia can result in endotoxic shock,

TABLE 2.13 Gram Negative Bacteria and Diseases Associated with These Microorganisms

Cell shape	Genus	Disease
Cocci	*Neisseriae*	Gonorrhea Meningitis
Rods	*Pseudomonas*	Wound, burn infection Pneumonia Eye infection
	Escherichia	Gastroenteritis Urinary tract infection
	Shigella	Dysentery
	Proteus	Urinary tract infection
	Hemophilus	Infantile meningitis Chronic bronchitis
	Salmonella	Typhoid fever Food poisoning
	Brucella	Animal infections

which is a common cause of morbidity and mortality in hospital patients. Detection of endotoxemia by the LAL test was first assessed by Fossard et al. in 1974 (105). They concluded that the LAL test is a simple, rapid, and reliable method for detecting endotoxemia. Early detection permits early and vigorous treatment of the infection in which the LAL test can be used to monitor the effectiveness of the treatment.

LAL assay found high plasma endotoxin levels in patients suffering from sepsis, malignant tumors, leukemia, and decompensated liver cirrhosis (106). A modification of the LAL test was required to eliminate interference factors located in platelet-rich plasma or serum. A simple addition of perchloric acid to plasma in a final concentration of 1.25% eliminated the inhibitors. LAL assay currently is being applied in studies trying to determine the correlation of endotoxin levels and various diseases.

Although not sanctioned by the FDA, the LAL test has proven to be very useful in the diagnosis of meningitis caused by pyrogenic radionuclide substances used in cisternography (107) and meningitis resulting from gram negative bacteria (108—111). The sensitivity, reliability, and rapidity of the LAL method are vitally important because of the serious toxicity problems associated with pyrogens and bacteria in CSF (112). The LAL test on CSF was found to be clinically useful in neonates suffering from gram negative infection (60).

The LAL test has been used successfully and holds important future applications in diagnosing and monitoring such various disease states as gingival inflammation (113), bacteriuria (114), postanasthia hepatitis (115), urinary tract infections (116), mastitic milk (117), gram negative sepsis resulting from burns (118), gonococcal cervicitis in women (119), and gonorrhea (120, 121).

Food

LAL testing has reached into some areas of food and drinking water processing. LAL has been used to determine endotoxin levels in drinking water (122, 123), marine environment (124), sugar (125), and ground beef (126). The levels of endotoxin provide evidence of the microbial quality of the food material. For example, LAL found ≤10 ng/g endotoxin for both white and beet raw sugar while 100 ng/g endotoxin was found in imported cane raw sugar (125).

Other Applications

The LAL test has proven to be a valuable test for the detection of endotoxin extracted from surgeons' sterile latex gloves (127) and operating nebulizers used in respiratory therapy (128).

Validation of dry heat sterilization and depyrogenation cycles based on the destruction of endotoxin can be accomplished through the employment of the LAL test (129, 130). This could not be accomplished practically using the USP rabbit test.

MODIFICATIONS OF RABBIT AND LAL TESTS FOR PYROGEN

Ultrafiltration, using a membrane having a fraction molecular weight of 10,000, has been used to separate endotoxin contamination from injectable solutions of sodium ampicillin (131). The filtrate solution contained endotoxin while the antibiotic remained entrapped on the filter. Samples of the filtrate were tested for pyrogenicity by the rabbit pyrogen test, the LAL gelation test, and the chromogenic assay method. All three tests were positive for endotoxin. Without ultrafiltration the presence of sodium ampicillin interferes with rabbit, LAL, and chromogenic detection of endotoxin (89). Ultrafiltration also allows concentration of endotoxin in drug preparations, facilitating detecting of minute (picogram) amounts of endotoxin.

REFERENCES

1. C. M. Good and H. E. Lane, Jr., The biochemistry of pyrogens, *Bull. Parenter. Drug Assoc.*, *31*, 116−120 (1977).
2. B. D. Davis, R. Dulbecco, H. N. Eisen, and H. S. Ginsberg, *Microbiology*, 3rd Edition, Harper and Row, Hagerstown, Maryland, 1981, p. 85.
3. E. Kenedi, H. Laburn, D. Mitchell, and F. P. Ross, On the pyrogenic action of intravenous lipid A in rabbits, *J. Physiol.*, *328*, 361−370 (1982).
4. T. Billroth, *Arch. Klin. Chir.*, *6*, 372 (1865).
5. J. Burion-Sanderson, On the process of fever, *Practitioner*, *16*, 257 (1876).
6. G. Roussy, *Gas. Hsp.*, Paris, *62*, 171 (1889).
7. E. Centanni, *Chem. Zbl.*, *6*, 587 (1894).
8. E. Hort and W. J. Penfold, *J. Hyg.*, *12*, 361 (1912), and *Proc. Roy. Soc. Med.*, Ser. B. *85*, 174 (1912).
9. J. L. Jona, *J. Hyg.*, *15*, 169 (1916).
10. R. Schmidt, *Muenchen Med. Wochenschr.*, *67*, 48 (1920).
11. F. B. Siebert, *Amer. J. Physiol.*, *67*, 90 (1923).
12. F. B. Siebert, The cause of many febrile reactions following intravenous injections, *Amer. J. Physiol.*, *71*, 621 (1924).

13. L. A. Rademacher, The causes of elimination of reactions after intravenous infusions, *Amer. Surg.*, *92*, 195 (1930).
14. H. D. CoTui and M. H. Schrift, Production of pyrogen by some bacteria, *J. Lab. Clin. Med.*, *27*, 569 (1942).
15. United States Pharmacopeia XXI/National Formulary XVI, Mack Publishing Co., Easton, Pannsylvania, 1985, pp. 1165—1167.
16. G. R. Peroneus, Pyrogen testing of parenteral pharmaceuticals, *Quality Control in the Pharmaceutical Industry* (M. Cooper, Ed.), Academic Press, New York, 1973.
17. C. J. Joubert, An automated temperature recording apparatus for the determination of pyrogens in intravenous solutions, *Lab. Anim.*, *14*, 103—106 (1980).
18. S. D. Greisman and R. B. Hornick, Comparative pyrogenic reactivity of rabbit and man to bacterial endotoxin, *Proc. Soc. Exp. Biol.*, N.Y., *131*, 1154—1158 (1969).
19. H. H. Freedman, Passive transfer of tolerance of pyrogenicity of bacterial endotoxin, *J. Exp. Med.*, *111*, 453—463 (1960).
20. D. L. Bornstein, C. Bradenberg, and W. Wood, Jr., Studies on the pathogenesis of fever XI: Quantitative features of the febrile response to leucocytic pyrogens, *J. Exp. Med.*, *117*, 349—364 (1963).
21. P. J. Weiss, Pyrogen testing, *J. Parenter. Drug Assoc.*, *32*, 236—241 (1978).
22. P. E. Mazur and M. D. McKendrick, Automated pyrogen testing system, *Pharm. Tech.*, *4*, 42—48 (1979).
23. *British Pharmacopoeia*, Volume II., Her Majesty's Stationery Office, London, 1980, pp. A153—154.
24. C. C. Mascoli and M. E. Weary, Limulus amebocyte lysate test for detecting pyrogens in parenteral injectable products and medical devices: Advantages to manufacturers and regulatory officials, *J. Parenter. Drug Assoc.*, *33*, 81—95 (1979).
25. R. Dabbath et al., Pyrogenicity of *E. coli* 055:B5 endotoxin by the USP rabbit test: A HIMA collaborative study, *J. Parenter. Drug Assoc.*, *34*, 212—216 (1980).
26. J. G. Dare and G. A. Mogey, Rabbit responses to human threshold doses of a bacterial pyrogen, *J. Pharm. Pharmacol.*, *6*, 325—332 (1954).
27. L. Bellentani, Cyclic and chronobiological considerations when employing the rabbit fever test, *Endotoxins and Their Detection with the Limulus Amebocyte Lysate Test* (S. W. Watson, J. Levin, and T. J. Novitsky, Eds.), Alan R. Liss, New York, 1982, pp. 329—342.

28. J. Levin and F. B. Bang, The role of endotoxin in the extracellular coagulation of Limulus blood, *Bull. Johns Hopkins Hosp.*, *115*, 265–274 (1964).

29. F. B. Bang, A bacterial disease of *Limulus polyphemus*, *Bull. Johns Hopkins Hosp.*, *98*, 325–351 (1956).

30. S. Marcus and J. R. Nelson, Tests alternative to the rabbit bioassay for pyrogens, *Dev. Biol. Stand.*, *34*, 45–55 (1977).

31. J. F. Cooper, H. D. Hochstein, and E. G. Seligman, The Limulus test for endotoxin (pyrogen) in radiopharmaceuticals and biologicals, *Bull. Parenter. Drug Assoc.*, *26*, 153–162 (1972).

32. J. F. Cooper, J. Levin, and H. N. Wagner, Jr., Quantitative comparison of *in vitro* and *in vivo* methods for the detection of endotoxin, *J. Lab. Clin. Med.*, *78*, 138–148 (1971).

33. J. F. Cooper and S. M. Pearson, Detection of endotoxin in biological products by the Limulus test, *Dev. Biol. Stand.*, *34*, 7–13 (1977).

34. *Federal Register*, *45*, 32299–32300 (1980).

35. T. Liu et al., Studies on the Limulus lysate coagulating system, *Biomedical Applications of the Horseshoe Crab (Limulidae)* (E. Cohen, Ed.), Alan R. Liss, New York, 1979, pp. 147–158.

36. T. Takagi et al., Amino acid sequence studies on horseshoe crab (*Tachypleus tridentatus*) coagulogen and the mechanism of gel formation, *Biomedical Applications of the Horseshoe Crab (Limulidae)* (E. Cohen, Ed.), Alan R. Liss, New York, 1979, pp. 169–184.

37. M. W. Mosesson et al., Structural studies of the coagulogen of amebocyte lysate for *Limulus polyphemus*, *Biomedical Applications of the Horseshoe Crab (Limulidae)* (E. Cohen, Ed.), Alan R. Liss, New York, 1979, pp. 159–168.

38. K. Tsuji and K. A. Steindler, Use of magnesium to increase sensitivity of *Limulus* amoebocyte lysate for detection of endotoxin, *Appl. Environ. Micro.*, *45*, 1342–1350 (1983).

39. J. F. Cooper and M. E. Neely, Validation of the LAL test for end product evaluation, *Pharm. Tech.*, *4*, 72–79 (1980).

40. J. F. Cooper, Principles and application of the Limulus test for pyrogen in parenteral drugs, *Bull. Parenter. Drug Assoc.*, *29*, 122–130 (1975).

41. H. D. Hochstein, The LAL test versus the rabbit pyrogen test for endotoxin detection, *Pharm. Tech.*, *5*, 37–42 (1981).

42. *Draft Guideline for Validation of Limulus Amebocyte Lysate Test as an End Product Endotoxin Test for Human and*

Animal Parenteral Drugs, Biological Products, and Medical Devices, Food and Drug Administration, February 2, 1983, pp. 33—34.

43. K. L. Melvaer and D. Fystro, Modified micromethod of the Limulus amoebocyte lysate assay for endotoxin, *Appl. Environ. Micro.*, *43*, 493—494 (1982).

44. J. H. Jorgensen and G. A. Alexander, Automation of the Limulus amoebocyte lysate test by using the Abbott MS-2 microbiology system, *Appl. Environ. Microbiol.*, *41*, 1316—1320 (1981).

45. T. J. Novitsky, S. S. Ryther, M. J. Case, and S. W. Watson, Automated LAL testing of parenteral drugs in the Abbott MS-2, *J. Parenter. Sci. Tech.*, *36*, 11—16 (1982).

46. J. H. Jorgensen and G. A. Alexander, Rapid detection of significant bacteriuria by use of an automated Limulus amoebocyte lysate assay, *J. Clin. Microbiol.*, *16*, 587—589 (1982).

47. B. Ditter et al., Detection of endotoxin in blood and other specimens by evaluation of photometrically registered LAL-reaction kinetics in microliter plates, *Endotoxins and Their Detection with the Limulus Amebocyte Lysate Test* (S. W. Watson, J. Levin, and T. J. Novitsky, Eds.), Alan R. Liss, New York, 1982, pp. 385—392.

48. M. Harada, T. Morita, and S. Iwanaza, A new assay method for bacterial endotoxins using horseshoe crab clotting enzyme, *J. Med. Enzymol.*, *3*, 43 (1978).

49. J. F. Cooper, Chromogenic substrates offer realistic alternative to LAL gel endpoint, *Partic. Micro. Contr.*, *2*, 32—33 (1983).

50. T. J. Novitsky, LAL methodology: The choice is yours, *Med. Dev. Diagn. Ind.*, Jan. 1984, pp. 49—53.

51. U.S. Food and Drug Administration, Licensing of Limulus amebocyte lysate: Use as an alternative for rabbit pyrogen test, *Federal Register*, *42*:57749 (1977).

52. Parenteral Drug Association, *Parenteral Drug Association Response to FDA Draft Guideline for the Use of Limulus Amebocyte Lysate*, Information Bulletin #3, March, 1980.

53. K. Tsuji, K. A. Steindler, and S. J. Harrison, *Limulus* amebocyte lysate assay for endotoxin for detection and quantitation of endotoxin in a small-volume parenteral product, *Appl. Environ. Micro.*, *40*, 533—538 (1980).

54. R. J. Elin and S. M. Wolff, Nonspecificity of the Limulus amebocyte lysate test: Positive reaction with polynucleotides and proteins, *J. Infect. Dis.*, *128*, 3 (1973).

55. J. D. Sullivan and S. W. Watson, Factors affecting the sensitivity of Limulus lysate, *Appl. Microbiol.*, *28*, 1023–1026 (1974).

56. H. J. Ronneberger, Comparison of the pyrogen tests in rabbits and with Limulus lysate, *Dev. Biol. Stand.*, *34*, 27–32 (1977).

57. G. Nyerges and S. Jaszovszky, Reliability of the rabbit pyrogen test and of the Limulus test in predicting the pyrogenicity of vaccines in man, *Acta Micro. Acad. Sci. Hung.*, *28*, 235–243 (1981).

58. R. E. Wachtel and K. Tsuji, Comparison of Limulus amebocyte lysates and correlation with the United States Pharmacopoeia pyrogen test, *Appl. Environ. Microbiol.*, *33*, 1265–1269 (1977).

59. C. W. Twohy, M. L. Nierman, A. P. Duran, and T. E. Munson, Comparison of Limulus amebocyte lysates from different manufacturers, *J. Parenter. Sci. Tech.*, *37*, 93–96 (1983).

60. M. C. Kelsey, A. P. Lipscomb and J. M. Mowles, Limulus amoebocyte lysate endotoxin test: An aid to the diagnosis in the septic neonate?, *J. Infection, 4*, 69–72 (1982).

61. A. Wildfeuer et al., Use of Limulus assay to compare the biological activity peptidoglycan and endotoxin, *A. Immutaetsforsch.*, *149*, 258–264 (1975).

62. K. Brunson and D. W. Watson, Limulus amebocyte lysate reaction with streptococcal pyrogenic endotoxin, *Infect. Immun.*, *14*, 1256–1258 (1970).

63. M. Suzuki et al., Gelation of Limulus lysate by synthetic dextran derivatives, *Microbiol. Immunol.*, *21*, 419–425 (1977).

64. D. H. Fine et al., Limulus lysate activity of lipoteichoic acids, *J. Dent. Res.*, *56*, 1500–1501 (1977).

65. M. Platica, W. Harding, and V. P. Hollander, Dithiols stimulate endotoxin in the Limulus reaction, *Experientia, 34*, 1154–1155 (1978).

66. F. C. Pearson and M. Weary, The significance of Limulus amebocyte lysate test specificity on the pyrogen evaluation of parenteral drugs, *J. Parenter. Drug Assoc.*, *34*, 103–108 (1980).

67. A. Gardi and G. Arpagaus, The Limulus amebocyte lysate test: A useful tool for the control of plasma fractions, *Dev. Biol. Stand.*, *34*, 21–26 (1977).

68. D. Fumarola and E. Jirillo, Limulus test, parenteral drugs and biological products: An approach, *Dev. Biol. Stand.*, *34*, 97–100 (1977).

69. C. C. Mascoli and M. E. Weary, Applications and advantages of the Limulus amebocyte lysate (LAL) pyrogen test for parenteral injectable products, *Prog. Clin. Biol. Res.*, *29*, 387–402 (1979).

70. M. Weary and B. Baker, Utilization of the Limulus amebocyte lysate test for pyrogen testing large-volume parenterals, administration sets, and medical devices, *Bull. Parenter. Drug Assoc.*, *31*, 127–133 (1977).

71. C. C. Mascoli, Limulus amebocyte lysate (LAL) test for detecting pyrogens in parenteral injectables and medical devices, *J. Pharm. Belg.*, *34*, 145–155 (1979).

72. J. VanNoordwijk and Y. DeJong, Comparison of the LAL test with the rabbit test: False positives and false negatives, *Dev. Biol. Stand.*, *34*, 39–43 (1977).

73. K. Z. McCullough and S. A. Scolnick, Effect of semisynthetic penicillins on the Limulus lysate test, *Antimicrob. Ag. Chemother.*, *9*, 856 (1976).

74. K. L. Smith, Sequential analysis applied to biological control tests for pharmacopoeia substances, *Quantitative Methods in Pharmacology* (J. deJonge, Ed.), North Holland, Amsterdam, 1961, pp. 49–55.

75. J. VanNoordwijk and Y. DeJong, Comparison of the Limulus test for endotoxin with the rabbit test for pyrogens of the European pharmacopoeia, *J. Biol. Stand.*, *4*, 131–139 (1976).

76. J. D. Sullivan and S. W. Watson, Inhibitory effect of heparin on the Limulus test for endotoxin, *J. Clin. Microbiol.*, *2*, 151 (1975).

77. J. D. Sullivan and S. W. Watson, Purification and properties of the clotting enzyme from Limulus lysate, *Biochem. Biophys. Res. Commun.*, *66*, 848–855 (1975).

78. A. K. Highsmith, R. L. Anderson, and J. R. Allen, Application of the Limulus amebocyte lysate assay in outbreaks of pyrogenic reaction associated with parenteral fluids and medical devices, *Endotoxins and Their Detection with the Limulus Amebocyte Lysate Test* (S. W. Watson, J. Levin, and T. J. Novitsky, Eds.), Alan R. Liss, New York, 1982, pp. 287–299.

79. C. A. DeMurphy and T. R. Aneiros, ^{99m}Tc-radiopharmaceuticals and the Limulus test, *J. Parenter. Drug Assoc.*, *34*, 268–271 (1980).

80. B. A. Rhodes and B. Y. Croft, *Basics of Radiopharmacy*, C. B. Mosby, St. Louis, Missouri, 1978, p. 81.

81. H. F. Oettgen et al., Toxicity of *E. coli* L-asparaginase in man, *Cancer*, *25*, 253–278 (1970).

82. D. Fumarola, Possible endotoxin contamination in some anti-tumor agent preparations: Study with the Limulus amebocyte lysate test II, *Farmaco, 32,* 444—448 (1977).
83. S. E. Siegel, R. Nachum, S. Leimbrock, and M. Karon, Detection of bacterial endotoxin in anti-tumor agents, *Cancer Trt. Reports., 60,* 9—15 (1976).
84. M. J. Case, S. S. Ryther, and T. J. Novitsky, Detection of endotoxin in antibiotic solutions with *Limulus* amoebocyte lysate, *Antimicro. Agents Chemother., 23,* 649—652 (1983).
85. R. Nandan and D. R. Brown, An improved *in vitro* pyrogen test to detect picograms of endotoxin contamination in intravenous fluids using Limulus amebocyte lysate, *J. Lab. Clin. Med., 89,* 910—918 (1977).
86. R. J. Guzman and H. Kuo, Pyrogen testing of an intravenous fat emulsion, *Prog. Clin. Biol. Res., 29,* 333—337 (1979).
87. S. L. Gaffin, Endotoxin determination in viscous opaque solutions of iron dextran by Limulus amebocyte lysate, *Prog. Clin. Biol. Res., 29,* 221—227 (1979).
88. S. J. Harrison, K. Tsuji, and R. M. Enzinger, Application of LAL for detection of endotoxin in antibiotic preparations, *Biomedical Applications of the Horseshoe Crab (Limulidae)* (E. Cohen, Ed.), Alan R. Liss, New York, 1979, pp. 353—365.
89. P. M. Newsome, Penicillins and the Limulus amebocyte lysate test for endotoxin, *J. Pharm. Pharmacol., 29,* 204—206 (1977).
90. I. L. Bennett, Jr., R. G. Petersdorf, and W. R. Keene, Pathogenesis of fever: Evidence for direct cerebral action of bacterial endotoxins, *Trans. Assoc. Amer. Phy., 70,* 64 (1957).
91. F. C. Pearson et al., Applications of the Limulus amebocyte lysate assay to testing of HSA: Symposium on sterilization microbiology,
92. H. Ronneberger, LAL assay for plasmaproteins, *Endotoxins and Their Detection with the Limulus Amebocyte Lysate Test* (S. W. Watson, J. Levin, and T. J. Novitsky, Eds.), Alan R. Liss, New York, 1982, pp. 261—267.
93. S. C. Rastogi, H. D. Hochstein, and E. G. Seligimann, Statistical determination of endotoxin content in influenze vaccine by the LAL test, *J. Clin. Microbiol., 2,* 144 (1977).
94. K. J. Johnson, P. A. Ward, S. Goralnick, and M. J. Osborn, Isolation from human serum of an inactivator of bacterial lipopolysaccharide, *Amer. J. Pathol., 88,* 559 (1977).

95. R. C. Skarnes, The inactivation of endotoxin after interaction with certain proteins of normal serum, *Ann. N.Y. Acad. Sci.*, *133*, 644–622 (1966).

96. F. S. Rosen, R. C. Skarnes, and M. Landy, Inactivation of endotoxin by humoral component III. Role of divalent cation and dialyzable component, *J. Exp. Med.*, *108*, 701 (1958).

97. J. Levin, The *Limulus* test and bacterial endotoxins: Some persepctives, *Endotoxins and Their Detection with the Limulus Amoebocyte Lysate Test* (S. W. Watson, J. Levin, and T. J. Novitsky, Eds.), Alan R. Liss, New York, 1982, pp. 7–24.

98. J. Levin, P. A. Tomasulo, and R. S. Oser, Detection of endotoxin in human blood and demonstration of an inhibitor, *J. Lab. Clin. Med.*, *75*, 903 (1970).

99. R. B. Reinhold and J. Fine, A technique of quantitative measurement of endotoxin in human plasma, *Proc. Soc. Exp. Biol. Med.*, *137*, 334 (1971).

100. M. S. Cooperstock, R. P. Tucker, and J. V. Baublis, Possible pathogenic role of endotoxin in Reye's syndrome, *Lancet*, *1*, 1272 (1975).

101. L. Baek, New, sensitive rocket immunoelectrophoretic assay for measurement of the reaction between endotoxin and *Limulus* amoebocyte lysate, *J. Clin. Micro.*, *17*, 1013–1020 (1983).

102. V. C. Ross, LAL testing of medical devices: A regulatory update, *Med. Dev. Diagn. Ind.*, March, 1984, 37–39, 91.

103. *Guidelines for the Use of Limulus Lysate Test (LAL) for Pyrogen Testing of Medical Devices*, HIMA Report No. 78-8, Health Industry Manufacturers Association, Washington, D.C., 1978.

104. *HIMA Collaborative Study for the Pyrogenicity Evaluation of a Reference Endotoxin by the USP Rabbit Test*, HIMA Document Series, *1*, No. 7, Health Industry Manufacturers Association, Washington, D.C., 1979.

105. D. P. Fossard, V. V. Kakkar, and P. A. Elsey, Assessment of Limulus test for detecting endotoxaemia, *Brit. Med. J.*, *2*, 465 (1974).

106. T. Obayashi et al., New Limulus amoebocyte lysate test for endotoxeamia, *Lancet*, *1*, 289 (1982).

107. J. F. Cooper and J. C. Harbert, Endotoxin as a cuase of aseptic meningitis after radionuclide cisternography, *J. Nuc. Med.*, *16*, 809–813 (1975).

108. J. H. Jorgensen and J. C. Lee, Rapid diagnosis of gram-negative bacterial meningitis by the Limulus endotoxin assay, *J. Clin. Microbiol.*, *7*, 12 (1978).

109. N. Clumeck, Limulus test and meningitis, *Brit. Med. J.*, *1*, 777 (1977).

110. D. Dyson and G. Cassady, Use of Limulus lysate for detecting gram-negative neonatal meningitis, *Pediatrics*, *58*, 105 (1976).

111. S. Ross et al., Limulus lysate test for gram-negative bacterial meningitis, *JAMA*, *233*, 1366 (1975).

112. G. H. McCracken and L. D. Sarff, Endotoxin in cerebrospinal fluid, *JAMA*, *235*, 617 (1976).

113. L. Shapiro et al., Endotoxin determinations in gingival inflammation, *J. Periodontal Res.*, *43*, 59 (1972).

114. S. H. Jorgensen et al., Rapid detection of gram-negative bacteriuria by use of the Limulus endotoxin assay, *J. App. Micro.*, *26*, 38—42 (1973).

115. C. Lomanto et al., Horseshoe crabs, endotoxemia and post-anesthesia hepatitis, *N.Y. State J. Med.*, Nov. 1974, 2145.

116. J. M. Jorgensen and P. M. Jones, Comparative evaluation of the Limulus assay and the direct gram stain for the detection of significant bacteriuria, *Amer. J. Clin. Pathol.*, *63*, 142 (1975).

117. G. Hartmann and A. Saran, Application of the Limulus amebocyte lysate test to the detection of gram-negative bacterial endotoxin in normal and mastitic milk, *Res. Vet. Sci.*, *20*, 342 (1976).

118. N. Harris and R. Feinstein, A new Limulus assay for the detection of endotoxin, *J. Trauma*, *17*, 714—718 (1977).

119. V. A. Spagna, R. B. Prior, and G. A. Sawaya, Sensitivity, specificity, and predictive values of the Limulus lysate assay for detection of exclusion of gonococcal cervicitis, *J. Clin. Micro.*, *16*, 77—81 (1982).

120. B. L. Hainer, P. Danylchuk, J. Cooper, and C. W. Weart, Limulus lysate assay in detection of gonorrhea in women from a low-incidence population, *Am. J. Obstet. Gynecol.*, *144*, 67—71 (1982).

121. V. A. Spagna and R. B. Prior, Detection of gonorrhea by Limulus lysate assay, *Am. J. Obstet. Bynecol.*, *146*, 474—475 (1983).

122. J. H. Jorgensen, J. C. Lee, and H. R. Pahren, Rapid detection of bacterial endotoxin in drinking water and renovated waste water, *J. Appl. Microbiol.*, *32*, 347—351 (1976).

123. T. M. Evans, J. E. Schillinger, and D. G. Stuart, Rapid determination of bacteriological water quality by using Limulus lysate, *Appl. Environ. Microbiol.*, *35*, 376–382 (1978).

124. S. W. Watson et al., Determination of bacterial number and biomass in the marine environment, *Appl. Environ. Microbiol.*, *33*, 940–946 (1977).

125. G. Haskae and R. Nystrand, Determination of endotoxins in sugar with the LAL test, *Appl. Environ. Microbiol.*, *38*, 1078–1080 (1979).

126. J. M. Jay, The Limulus lysate endotoxin assay as a test of microbial quality of ground beef, *J. Appl. Bacteriol.*, *43*, 99–109 (1977).

127. R. Kure, H. Grendahl, and J. Paulssen, Pyrogens from surgeons' sterile latex gloves, *Acta Path. Microbiol. Immunol. Scand. Sect. B*, *90*, 85–88 (1982).

128. D. J. Reinhardt et al., LAL and direct sampling methods for surveillance of operating nebulizers, *Appl. Environ. Microbiol.*, *42*, 850–855 (1981).

129. M. J. Akers, K. M. Ketron, and B. R. Thompson, F value requirements for the destruction of endotoxin in the validation of dry heat sterilization/depyrogenation cycles, *J. Parenteral Sci. Tech.*, *36*, 23–27 (1982).

130. K. Tsuji and S. J. Harrison, Dry heat destruction of lipopolysaccharide: Dry heat destruction kinetics, *Appl. Environ. Microbiol.*, *36*, 710 (1978).

131. S. Takahashi, S. Yano, Y. Nagaoka, K. Kawamura, and S. Minami, A highly sensitive pyrogen test for antibiotics I: Detection of trace amounts of endotoxin in injectable sodium ampicillin preparations, *J. Pharm. Sci.*, *72*, 739–742 (1983).

3
Particulate Matter Testing

INTRODUCTION

No quality control test, parenteral or non-parenteral, can cause
more frustration for quality control authorities than inspection of
injectable solutions for the presence of particulate matter. The
oldest, yet most commonly used test for particulate matter evaluation involves human visual examination. Such examination is subjective, time-consuming, and limited in the types of parenteral
products and containers that can be inspected. This has stimulated
many studies regarding ways of not only improving efficiency of
human inspection but also developing and improving methods of
detecting particulate matter electronically.

The United States Pharmacopeia (USP) requirement for injectable products specifies that "each final container of injection be subjected individually to a physical inspection, whenever the nature
of the container permits, and that every container whose contents
show evidence of contamination with visible foreign material be rejected" (1). Additional specifications are required for particulate matter content and analysis in large-volume injections for
single-dose infusion (2). For the 21st edition of the USP, specifications have been written for particulate matter limits in small-
volume parenterals.

Why are injectable products to be free of visible evidence of particulate matter? Primarily, lack of particulate matter conveys a

clean, quality product, indicative of the high quality standards employed by the product manufacturer. Moreover, in recent years, particulate matter has become known as a potential hazard to the safety of the patient undergoing parenteral therapy. While there still seems to be a lack of sufficient clinical data to incriminate particles as producers of significant clinical complications during parenteral therapy, it is a universal belief in the health care field that particulate matter does present a clinical hazard and must be absent from the injectable solution.

The aim of this chapter is to concentrate on current and future particle testing methods in the quality control analysis of parenteral solutions. Two primary methods of particle analysis—visual inspection and electronic particle counting—will be discussed in detail. Groves' textbook (3) has been used as a major resource of information contained in several of the sections of this chapter.

BACKGROUND OF PARTICULATE MATTER
CONCERNS IN PARENTERAL PRODUCTS

It is interesting to realize that all the attention given today to the problems and analysis of particulate matter in parenteral products did not exist before the 1940s. After the inclusion of the first injectable product in the USP (12th edition) in 1942, Godding (4) was the first individual to publish an article concerning the need for standards in the visual inspection of particulate matter. The 13th edition of the USP (5) gave a detailed method for inspecting an injectable solution against a white and black background using a light intensity between 100 and 350 footcandles at a distance of 10 inches. Interestingly, the method described in the 13th edition is still widely used in manual inspections for evidence of visible particulate matter.

The "rule-of-thumb" standard that a person with 20/20 vision under inspection conditions should be able to detect particles having sizes of approximately 50 μm came from a report by Brewer and Dunning (6). This detection limit has persevered since 1957 although recent research suggests that inspectors should actually be able to see particles in the size range of 20 μm (7).

In the early 1950s a number of reports began citing evidence of biological hazards produced by foreign injected materials. Among the materials found to cause pulmonary granulomata or emboli were cotton fibers (8) and cellulose (9). Glass particles and their potential hazard was studied by Brewer and Dunning (6) and later by Gradinger (10), but no evidence of foreign body reactions in animals were found. These and other reports led to the classic work done by Garvan and Gunner published in 1963 and 1964 (11, 12). These Australian physicians showed that foreign body granulomas could be produced experimentally in the lungs of rabbits following the administration of 500 ml saline solution contaminated with visible particulate matter. Most commercial intravenous solutions inspected contained particle contamination and the source of most of the particles was attributed to the rubber closure. For every 500 ml of particle-contaminated intravenous solution injected into a rabbit, 5000 granulomas appeared in the lungs. Garvan and Gunner further found that similar granulomas appeared in the postmorten examinations of the lungs of patients receiving large volumes of intravenous fluids. Their comments included the possibility that postoperative pulmonary infarction was a result of particulate thrombosis. The repercussions of Garvan and Gunner's reports have stimulated numerous studies on the analysis and potential clinical hazards of particulate matter that continue to this day.

A collaborative study conducted by the Pharmaceutical Manufacturers Association (13) involved the intravenous injection of varying quantities and sizes of inert polystyrene spheres into hundreds of rats, then performing necropsies at various periods of time from one hour to 28 days following injection. The results were as follows:

1. Thirteen of 18 rats injected with 8×10^6 particles per kg at a particle size of 40 μm died within five minutes.
2. Rats showed normal blood studies, organ weights, and pathologic criteria after being injected with either 8×10^6 particle size 0.4 to 10 μm or 4×10^5 particles per kg of particle size 40 μm.
3. Particles in the 4 μm size range were found in the lung, liver, and spleen.
4. Particles in the 10 μm size range were found in the lung primarily, although particles were found in five other organs.
5. Particles in the 40 μm size range were found in the lungs and myocardial tissue.

It was concluded that non-reactive particles administered intravenously over a broad size range and up to dosages that produced death were without clinical or tissue toxicity. Much disagreement resulted over this conclusion, especially because of the artificial nature of the type of particle studied. However, the same size-dependent localization of particles in different organs was found in the case of glass particles derived from breaking the necks of glass ampuls (14). Large particles (> 20 μm) were retained mostly in the lungs of mice while smaller particles (5-10 μm) were found in the liver, spleen, and kidney. No glass particle was found in the brain.

The potential hazard of particulate matter has been implied in a number of reports, two of which are cited here. In a study of 173 patients undergoing cardiac catherization and/or surgery, 14 (8%) had fiber emboli in routine autopsy sections (15). The embolized fiber often resulted in narrowing or occlusion of the involved blood vessel. Three cases of myocardial infarction were associated with embolic fibers. Fibers were believed to have originated from various materials used in surgery and from drug solutions. It was concluded that particulate matter is a hazard and all steps must be taken to prevent its inadvertent administration.

A second critical report implicating the hazards of particulate matter was the work published by DeLuca et al. (16). In a repeated double-blind study of 146 patients, a significant reduction in the incidence of infusion phlebitis was seen when patients were administered intravenous fluids filtered through an in-line 0.45 μm filter. Other studies as reviewed by Turco and King (17) have supported this finding.

Particles greater than 7 μm in diameter are viewed to be more threatening than particles of smaller size (18). Pulmonary capillaries are approximately 7 μm in diameter. Thus, theoretically, a particle greater than 7 μm can be trapped in the vascular bed, resulting in multiple pulmonary infarctions.

Freedom from visible evidence of particulate matter is a basic, essential characteristic of injectable products. Such a characteristic imparts three significant qualities to the product:

1. Significance to the manufacturer—lack of particulate matter indicates good production technique and a quality product.
2. Significance to the user—lack of particulate matter indicates a clean product that is safe to the patient, and conveys high quality standards employed by the manufacturer of the product.
3. Clinical significance—lack of particulate matter indicates the lack of potential hazards resulting from particles entering the circulatory system, although controversy still exists regarding the hazards of particulate matter (19).

NATURE AND SOURCE OF PARTICULATES

Anything that directly or indirectly comes in contact with a parenteral solution, including the solvent and solutes composing the solution itself, represents a potential source of particulate contamination. Table 3.1 lists common sources of particulates found in parenteral solutions.

The type and approximate size range of particulates found in parenteral products are listed in Table 3.2. The smallest capillary blood vessels are considered to have a diameter of approximately 5 μm. Thus, all particles having a size equal to or greater than 5 μm can conceivably become entrapped in and occlude a blood capillary. Most particulates, as seen in Table 3.2, potentially can be

TABLE 3.1   Common Sources of Particulate Matter

1. Chemicals

    a. Undissolved substances
    b. Trace contaminants

2. Solvent impurities

3. Packaging components

    a. Glass
    b. Plastic
    c. Rubber
    d. I.V. administration sets

4. Environmental contaminants

    a. Air
    b. Surfaces
    c. Insect parts

5. Processing equipment

    a. Glass
    b. Stainless steel
    c. Rubber
    d. Rust

6. Filter fibers

7. People

    a. Skin
    b. Hair
    c. Gowning

TABLE 3.2 Type and Approximate Size Range of Some Extraneous Materials Reported in Parenteral Solutions

Material	Approximate size range (μm)
Glass	1
Metal	1
Rubber	1 to 500
Starch	1
Zinc oxide	1
Whiting	1
Carbon black	1
Clay	1
Diatoms	1 to 5
Bacteria	2
Fungi and fungal spores	20
Insect parts	20
Cellulose fibers	1 to 100
Trichomes	10
Miscellaneous crystalline material	1
Talc	1
Asbestos fibers	1 to 100
Unidentified fibers	1

Source: Ref. 3.

this size and, obviously, represent a hazard to the health of a patient administered parenteral medications containing these contaminants.

It seems that regardless of whatever painstaking procedures are undertaken to eliminate particle contamination, parenteral solutions always contain a certain degree of particulate matter. It is always an uncertainty whether the particles originated during the manufacturing and packaging process or were introduced during the analysis of the solution for the presence of particulates. The emphasis on technique in the analysis of particulate matter has been stressed by Draftz and Graf (20) and McCrone (21). It is imperative that particles seen in solutions not have originated during the particle measurement and identification procedures.

PARTICULATE MATTER STANDARDS

The first reference to particulate matter in the USP occurred in the eighth edition in 1905 (22, 23). Diphtheria Antitoxin, a hypodermic injection product, was described as a "transparent or slightly turbid liquid." Not until 1936, in the National Formulary (NF), sixth edition, was the term "clearness" defined for parenteral products (24): "Aqueous Ampul Solutions are to be clear; i.e., when observed over a bright light, they shall be substantially free from precipitate, cloudiness or turbidity, specks or fibers, or cotton hairs, or any undissolved material."

The words "substantially free" caused interpretative difficulties; thus, in 1942, the NF, seventh edition, provided a definition: ". . . substantially free shall be construed to mean a preparation which is free from foreign bodies that would be readily discernible by the unaided eye when viewed through a light reflected from a 100-watt mazda lamp using as a medium a ground glass and a background of black and white." It was also in 1942 that the 12th edition of the USP contained its first particulate matter standard:

Appearance of Solution or Suspension Injections which are solutions of soluble medicaments must be clear, and free (note the absence of "substantially") of any turbidity or undissolved material which can be detected readily without magnification when the solution is examined against black and white backgrounds with a bright light reflected from a 100-watt mazda lamp or its equivalent.

The requirement that every injectable product in its final container be subjected individually to visual inspection appeared in the eighth edition of the USP (5). This requirement has remained essentially unchanged; as the twenty-first edition states: "Good pharmaceutical practice requires also that each final container of injection be subjected individually to a physical inspection, whenever the nature of the container permits, and that every container whose contents show evidence of contamination with visible foreign material be rejected" (1).

The problem with the above USP statement lies with the word "visible." Visible has the connotation of particles being seen with the unaided eye. The unaided eye can discern, at best, particles at sizes of about 40-50 μm. Detection of smaller particles cannot be accomplished assuredly with the USP physical inspection test. Health care professionals became increasingly concerned about the aspect of intravenous solutions, especially large-volume parenterals, contaminated with particles too small to be seen with the unaided eye, yet still hazardous when introduced into the veins of a recumbant patient. In the middle 1970s the USP and FDA co-sponsored the establishment of the National Coordinating Committee on Large-Volume Parenterals (NCCLVP). The NCCLVP then established a subcommittee on methods of testing for particulate matter in LVPs. Ultimately, the efforts of this subcommittee resulted in the establishment of the USP microscopic assay procedure for the determination of particulate matter in LVPs for single-dose infusion and set upper limit acceptable particle standards at particle standards at particle sizes of 10 μm and 25 μm (25).

The USP standards for LVPs came after standards were first established in Australia and Britain. The Australian standards were based on the research by Vessey and Kendall (26) and their results are reported in Table 3.3 along with the upper limit particle specifications in the British Pharmacopoeia (BP) and USP.

Because of the widespread acceptance of instrumental methods for counting and sizing particles, several alternatives to the present

TABLE 3.3 Particulate Matter Standards in Various Compendia Compared to Those Suggested by Vessey and Kendall

Particle size (≥μm)	Vessey and Kendall (26)	Australia[a] (27)	British Pharmacopoeia[b] (28)	U. S. Pharmacopeia[c] (2)
2	1000	−	1000 (500)	−
3.5	250	−	−	−
5	100	100	100 (80)	−
10	25	−	−	50
20	−	2	−	−
25	−	−	−	5

[a]Mean count of at least 10 containers using light-blockage method. See text for additional specifications.
[b]Particle standards apply only to specific solutions using conductivity (Coulter Counter). Numbers in parentheses refer to particle limits if light blockage (HIAC) is used.
[c]Particle standards apply only to large-volume parenterals. Particle numbers and size determined by microscopic methods unless electronic methods have been shown to have equivalent reliability.

LVP particle limit specifications seen in Table 3.3 have been proposed. The National Biological Standards Laboratory (NBSL) of
Australia has adopted an approach that depends on the mean and
standard deviation of the results from 10 individual containers.
This approach takes into account the usually wide variation in par-
tical counts measured from container to container. As seen in
Table 3.3, under the Australian standards, no more than 100 and
2 particles per ml at particle sizes of 5 μm and 20 μm, respectively,
are permitted in LVP solutions. However, the Australian standards
also state that at the 5 μm particle size level, the sum of the mean
and twice the standard deviation is not more than 200; that is,

$$\bar{x} + 2s \leqslant 200$$

and at the 20 μm size, the sum of the mean particle count and twice
the standard deviation is not more than 4

$$\bar{x} + 2s \leqslant 4.$$

The Australian approach combines the mean values of 10 containers. Hailey et al. (29) suggested the use of a statistical limit that
would account for the mean and standard deviation of particle
counts obtained for *each* of the 10 containers tested. Their proposal uses a term called statistic S_T which is defined mathematically
as

$$S_T = [\Sigma(\bar{x} - T)^2/n]^{\frac{1}{2}}$$

where $\bar{x}$ is the mean value of n results and T is the target value
(the desired value of the system being measured). For LVPs, the
desired value would be zero (no particles) so the above equation
would become

$$S_T = [\Sigma\bar{x}^2/n]^{\frac{1}{2}}$$
$$S_T = [S^2(n - 1)/n + \bar{x}^2]^{\frac{1}{2}}$$

where S is the standard deviation. The advantage of the S_T
approach over the Australian draft standard is the increased
stringency of the S_T requirement on samples near the limit for
mean particle count and having large standard deviation. For
example, if $\bar{x}$ for 10 containers were 100.0, $\bar{x}$ + 2s were 134.4,
and S_T were 101.3, the sample would pass the Australian test

($\bar{x}$ + 2s less than 200) but fail the S_T test (value $\geq$ 100). The disadvantage of the S_T test is that it is based on a target of zero, a
level of cleanliness that can never be achieved. However, to use
any other target value would introduce additional problems as discussed by Hailey et al. (29). The authors conclude by stating that
an S_T target of zero does not add unrealistic constraints on manufacturers, but it does reduce the risk of passing a lot of LVP solution having a few containers that are extremely contaminated with
particles.

Groves (30, 31) has proposed that a single numerical value, the
index of contamination (C), be adopted as a standard for accepting
or rejecting LVP fluids. C is obtained from log particle size-log
particle number plots of solutions measured by Coulter Counter and
light blockage methods in which the results cross over at a size
threshold of around 6.0 μm. Using the log-log relationship for the
BP limits between 2 μm and 5 μm and extended the line to 6.0 μm,
the extrapolated number of particles equals 63.244. From previous
derivations outlined by Groves and Wana (31), the index of contamination may then be defined as

$$C = (\ln N_{1.0} - \ln 63.244)/m$$

where $N_{1.0}$ is the estimated number of particles per unit volume at
a size threshold of 1.0 μm and m is the slope of the particle size-
number distribution. This index has the advantage over the BP
limit tests in that it is not affected by the type of instrumental principle used to determine the parameters of the size distribution (see
the sections "Electronic Particle Counters" and "Comparison of
Microscopic and Electronic Particle Counting Methods" later in this
chapter). In addition, C can be calculated from data acquired at
size thresholds that do not necessarily coincide with those of the
BP tests, and calculations of C can be made readily and routinely
using on-line computerized quality control procedures.

VISUAL INSPECTION: MANUAL METHODS

Manual inspection by human inspectors for the presence of visible
particulate matter in parenteral solutions still remains the most
widely used particle test method. While electronic television mon-
itors have made significant strides in replacing 100% human inspection, the latter remains standard practice for end-product particle
analysis of parenteral products.

Each final container of a parenteral product should be inspected by a trained individual. Any evidence of visible particulate matter or other product/container defect provides the grounds for rejecting that container.

The Task Group No. 3 of the Parenteral Drug Association published guidelines to be considered in the design and evaluation of visual inspection procedures (32). These guidelines will be discussed in this section.

Equipment

Lighting may be fluorescent, incandescent, spot, and/or polarized. The most common source of light is fluorescent. The light source may be positioned above, below, or behind the units being inspected. The range of light intensity may vary between 100 and 350 footcandles. This intensity can be achieved either with one 100-watt, inside-frosted incandescent light bulb, or with three 15-watt fluorescent bulbs with the container held 10 inches from the light source. Certain types of products (e.g., colored solutions) or certain types of containers (e.g., amber) require increased light intensity over that normally used. As light intensity begins to weaken, due to age or usage, lamps should be replaced. Good practice demands that inspection lamps be monitored periodically.

A white and black background lighted with non-glaring light is the standard environment used for visual inspection of product containers. The white background aids in the detection of dark-colored particles. Light or refractile particles will appear against the black background.

Many manufacturers have progressed to the use of automated inspection equipment. Appropriate inspection procedure should specify and monitor the adjustment of the machine's operating parameters required to achieve a quality of inspection that is at least equivalent to that resulting from a previously established manual inspection procedure. Automated inspection machinery will be discussed in the following, "Visual Inspection: Automatic Methods."

A standard inspection booth contains an all-black interior except for the front entrance for the inspector. A vertical screen in the back of the booth is half black and half white. Light usually is projected vertically with frontal blockage to protect the observer's eyes from direct illumination. A magnifying lens at 2.5 × magnification may be set at eye level to aid the inspector in viewing the container in front of the white/black background. Excellent viewing is provided without distraction, and acuteness of vision is increased to improve the level of discrimination. It could be argued that the level of discrimination becomes too high, that is, containers are rejected that would not have been rejected had no magnification been used.

Inspection cabinets should have black side walls with a baffle to prevent the light source from impinging on the inspector's eye. Fluorescent lamps provide a better light source because these are more diffuse than incandescent lamps.

Methodology

Most inspection processes are referred to as off-line inspections, in which the inspection procedure occurs at the completion of the manufacturing, filling, and sealing process. In-line inspection of container components can also be done, especially if the production process can be suitably adapted to achieve the desired results without increasing the risk of microbial and particulate contamination. Obviously, the removal of defective containers, such as those showing cracks or the presence of particles, prior to the filling of the product assures product quality and minimizes loss of expensive drug products.

Standard operating procedures for inspection of parenteral containers depend on the kind of container inspected, that is, procedures will be slightly different for ampuls than for large-volume glass bottles, for amber vials than for flint vials, and for plastic bags than for glass containers. However, a basic procedure can be followed regardless of the type or size of container, and an example of such a procedure is given in Table 3.4.

Personnel

The human inspector determines the quality and success of the manual inspection process. Since the inspection process is subjective in nature, the main limitation of the process lies with restriction in the vision, attitude, and training of the individual inspector.

As a minimum standard, personnel assigned as inspectors should have good vision, corrected, if necessary, to acceptable standards. Inspectors should not be color-blind. Visual acuity should be tested at least on an annual basis.

Good attitude and concentration cannot be overemphasized. One of the major limitations of human inspection for particulate matter is reduced efficiency of the individual because of a lack of concentration. This can easily occur if the inspector suffers from extreme worry or other distraction resulting from outside personal pressures. Obviously, emotional stability is an important criterion in selecting inspectors.

TABLE 3.4 Basic Procedure for Manually Inspecting Clear
Solutions for Visible Evidence of Particulate Matter

1. Container of parenteral solution must be free of attached
   labels and thoroughly cleaned. Use a dampened non-linting
   cloth or sponge to remove external particles.

2. Hold container by its top and carefully swirl contents by
   rotating the wrist to start contents of the container moving in
   a circular motion. Vigorous swirling will create air bubbles,
   which should be avoided. Air bubbles will rise to the surface
   of the liquid; this helps to differentiate them from particulate
   matter.

3. Hold the container horizontally about 4 inches below the light
   source against a white and black background. Light should
   be directed away from the eyes of the inspector and hands
   should be kept from under the light source to prevent glare.

4. If no particles are seen, invert the container slowly and
   observe for heavy particles that may not have been suspended
   by swirling.

5. Reject any container having visible particles at any time
   during the inspection process.

Fatigue also becomes a major limitation of human inspection. Personnel should be provided appropriate relief from the inspection
function by rotating jobs and allowing for rest periods.

Formal training programs must precede the acceptance of an individual as a qualified inspector. The training program should include samples of both acceptable and unacceptable product containers that must be distinguished by the trainee. During the training
period all units inspected by the trainee should be re-inspected by
qualified inspectors to assure the quality of the inspection and the
development of the trainee. After the inspector has passed his/her
training period, performance tests should be done at random intervals to assure that quality standards are being maintained.

Two reports have been published concerning the effect of personnel experience on detection of particles in ampuls. Graham et al.
(33) found that inspectors with no experience and inspectors having at least 10 years experience agreed 64 to 83% of the time with
ampuls inspected under various conditions. Experienced inspectors
were faster in the inspection process. Baldwin et al. (34) found
that experienced inspectors reject ampuls at a greater rate (28.3%)

than did non-experienced inspectors (13.2%). Discrimination in particle detection apparently correlates with training and experience.

Comparison to Other Particle Inspection Methods

Manual visual inspection often is criticized because of its apparent inconsistency and unreliability. Its subjective nature, depending upon the judgment of uncontrolled and variable human evaluation of what may or may not be seen, drives many quality control specialists to seek other methods for achieving the same purpose— 100% non-destructure inspection of parenteral products for the presence of particulate matter.

Manual inspection can be compared to automatic electronic inspection methods on the basis of precision and accuracy (35). Precision is related to consistency, which measures the capability of any given process to detect the same conditions in repeated blind tests. Accuracy relates to bias, based on inequality of reject rates. When the precision and accuracy of manual inspection were compared to those demonstrated by Autoskan, an electronic video particulate inspection machine [see the section "Autoskan System" on page 60] two interesting conclusions were drawn:

1. Consistency of both methods, based on Cohen's Kappa statistic, were comparable. Autoskan was not superior to manual inspection in terms of repeatedly rejecting those ampuls containing particles.
2. Based on Cochran's Q statistic, bias was a problem with human inspection while appropriate settings of the Autoskan could eliminate machine bias. However, rejection rates were established using only one machine, while eight inspectors were tested and compared for their rejection rates of the same batched of ampul products. An example of rejection rates comparing machine and human inspectors is given in Table 3.5.

Reproducibility in human visual inspection was the subject of a paper by Faesen (36). Each of 1000 diamond-numbered ampuls and vials was inspected by 10 different inspectors, twice for each operator, using a Liquid Viewer, an inspection cabinet, and a Rota Ampul Inspection Machine (for ampuls only). The total number of rejects was registered following 60 inspections for the 1000 ampuls (three inspection methods performed twice) and 40 inspections for the 1000 vials (two inspection methods performed twice). Results indicated that reproducibility in visual inspection was nearly twice as high when performed with a Liquid Viewer as compared with

TABLE 3.5   Reject Rates for Four Products Inspected for
Particulate Matter by Autoskan and Eight Human Inspectors

| Product | Autoskan | Eight human inspectors | |
		Average	Range
A	22.2%	25.2%	19.7-29.2%
B	20.2%	21.5%	17.5-24.0%
C	20.3%	17.4%	15.5-19.5%
D	7.2%	7.9%	5.6-10.0%

Source: Ref. 35.

those performed with the inspection cabinet. For ampuls the value
reached using the Ampul Inspection Machine was less than 10% units
higher than that with the inspection cabinet. The Liquid Viewer
appeared to be the superior instrument for visually inspecting pa-
rentersl solutions.

In a panel discussion of mechanical inspection of ampuls (37-39),
it was stated that the average reject rate for ampuls inspected manually was 2-2.5%. Three inspection machines were compared to
manual inspection. Autoskan equipment (37) showed a reject rate
of 14.1%, the Rota Machine (38) increased the reject rate 0.5—1.5%
over that for manual inspection, and the Strunck Machine (39)
yielded a reject rate of 2.98%. The major advantage of machine inspection was simply their substantial increase in the number of
containers inspected per unit time.

Blanchard et al. (40) compared the human visual examination
method with several other methods for detection of particulate matter in large-volume parenteral solutions. Visual methods using
either the naked eye under diffuse light or a 2.5 copter lens
under diffuse light proved to be inadequate to other methods
(light scattering, Prototron, and microscopic examination after
filtration) in terms of sensitivity to low levels of particulate contamination. Not surprisingly, the visual methods showed a high
degree of subjectivity.

Visible Particle Sizes to the Unaided Eye

Since the number and size of particles in parenteral solutions have
become important characteristics to evaluate, it has been assumed

TABLE 3.6   Size of Particles of Varying Probability Levels[a]

Particle concentration	Particle size (μm) 50% chance	Particle size (μm) 100% chance
USP limit 50 particles/ml[b]	18.82	51.45
USP limit 5 particles/ml[c]	19.96	54.88
1-ml ampul, 1 particle	20.07	55.21
2-ml ampul, 1 particle	20.08	55.25
5-ml ampul, 1 particle	20.09	55.28
10-ml ampul, 1 particle	20.10	55.29
20-ml ampul, 1 particle	20.10	55.29
50-ml vial, 1 particle	20.10	55.29
1-liter large volume, 1 particle	20.10	55.29

[a]Arcsin $\sqrt{P_r}$ = 0.33689252 + 0.02231515 size + 0.000035 size vs. concentration −0.00008694 concentration.
[b]Not more than 50 particles/ml equal to or larger than 10 μm.
[c]Not more than 5 particles/ml equal to or larger than 10 μm.
Source: Ref. 7.

that particles larger than 40 or 50 μm are detectable by the unaided eye. Thus, in complying with USP requirements that any container showing visible evidence of particulate matter be rejected, it must be assumed that the average inspector will pass those solutions containing particles with a size $\leqslant$40 μm. This, of course, presents some discomfort for those who believe that particulate matter, especially in the size range of 10−40 μm, is clinically hazardous.

It is not only the size, but also, and probably more importantly, the number of large particles injected into man intravenously that is considered dangerous. Thus, official standards have been enforced for maximum allowable numbers of certain-sized particles in large-volume parenteral solutions (see the section "USP Test for Particulate Matter in Large-Volume Injections for Single-Dose Infusion"). Particulate contamination of sub-visible particles in small-volume parenterals, while bothersome to concerned health care professionals, has not presented as great a threat to human health and safety.

At least one attempt has been made to quantify the size and concentration of particles that can be detected by the unaided eye (7). Five milliliter ampuls containing 10 to 500 particles per ml of particle sizes between 5 and 40 μm (using polystyrene beads) were inspected by 17 inspectors in a standard booth. Based on a multiple linear analysis model that calculated the probability of rejecting an ampul as a function of particle size and concentration, sizes of particles detected at various concentration levels at 50% and 100% probability of rejection rates were predicted. These data are reproduced in Table 3.6. The authors concluded that a 50% probability of rejection rate be achieved with 20 μm particles in sample solutions in order for potential inspectors to be qualified for in-line inspection. However, it is interesting to note that a minimum particle size of 55 μm was required for all inspectors to reject all solutions containing this size of particle.

VISUAL INSPECTION: AUTOMATIC METHODS

Introduction

Manual visual inspection continues to be the most commonly used quality control method for particle detection in parenteral products. The limitations of depending on human inspection for rejecting particle-contaminated solutions have already been addressed. High technology strives for sophisticated automatic methodology to replace the dependency on human manual inspection. One area of high technology application to particle analysis in parenteral products is the development and improvement of electronic particle counters. The main limitation in the use of these instruments in particulate matter analyses resides in the fact that the tests are destructive. One hundred per cent inspection of each final container of parenteral product cannot be accomplished with electronic particle counters. The same limitation holds true for automated microscopic methods. The area of technology that offers the greatest potential for replacing human examination in 100% container inspection requirements is the area of computer-controlled, automatic electro-optic systems. Such systems are rapid, non-destructive, and reproducible in their inspection of parenteral products for foreign matter.

Early attempts to automate the 100% inspection process were reviewed by Groves (3). Systems developed and tested included the Brevetti device (41), Strunck machine (42), and the RCA machine (43). Despite considerable electronic ingenuity, all of these systems required human intervention at some stage of the inspection process, although Groves admitted this may be a consolation.

Hamlin et al. (44) were among the first investigators to test the use of television (TV) as an inspection device in detecting subvisible particulate matter. However, their main emphasis in using TV monitoring was as a research tool in detecting particles of 10 μm in experimental formulations for prediction of estimated shelf life based on physical stability. Also, TV monitoring required human involvement in viewing and rejecting particle contaminated solutions.

Technology has made significant improvements in fully automated parenteral product inspection procedures. Disadvantages of earlier automated systems, such as lack of standardization of performance, separating marks on the outer container surface from particles inside, failures to detect underfills or empty containers, and machine variabilities, have largely been eliminated with the automated systems available today.

Video inspection employs one of two basic mechanisms for automated container inspection (45). One mechanism uses imaging optics in which the particles suspended in the solution are illuminated by a fiber optic light system and imaged on a video display. These systems will be discussed in the section "Automated USP Particulate Matter Test" on page 176. The other mechanism employed in automated video inspection is based on light scattering from particulate matter, which is then received by a detection system and projected onto a television camera system. Several systems commercially available employ the light-scattering principle for automated video inspection. Among the most widely used systems are the Autoskan system, the Eisai AIM system, and the Schering PDS/A-V system. The prototron system (46, 47) at one time was a widely used non-destructive inspection method using laser light, but is no longer used today.

Autoskan System

The Autoskan system uses white light—in contrast to laser light, which is used by the Prototron system—to illuminate particles suspended in parenteral solutions. Particles will scatter the light, which is received by a television camera system. Any solution that contains particles will generate an error signal. That product container will not be released by the Autoskan system at the Accept station. Containers are also automatically rejected if they are either underfilled or overfilled.

Autoskan became the first totally automatic inspection system developed to detect particulate matter in injectable solutions. The instrument is suitable for the inspection of vials, ampuls, cartridges, and syringes. In Figure 3.1, ampuls on a rotary feed table are fed into the turret. The turret picks up the ampuls and intermittently transports them around to the inspection station where the lens of the television camera is located. The ampul is magnified by high-intensity light from below the check holding the ampul (see Figure 3.2). This light reflects particles moving in the liquid, making them visible to the camera (often visible also to the human eye). The Autoskan checks in the turret container motors that spin each container at an adjustable speed until the container comes before the lens of the television camera. The spinning is designed to

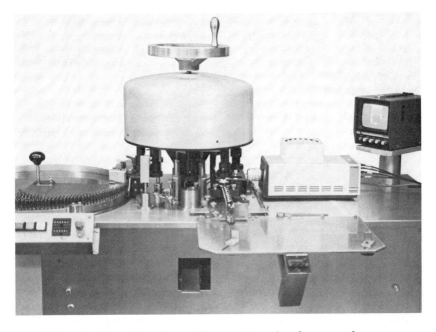

FIGURE 3.1 Autoskan inspection system showing ampuls on a rotary feed table leading into and exiting from the detection area. (Courtesy of the Lakso Company, Leominster, Pennsylvania.)

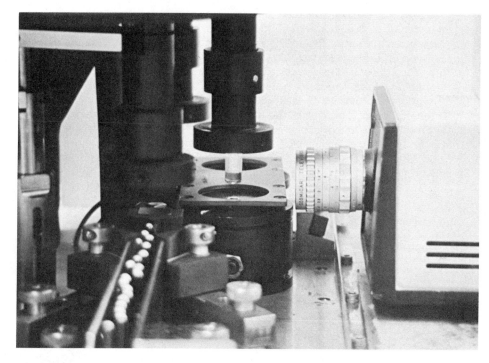

FIGURE 3.2   Close-up of ampul being inspected for particles by
the Autoskan system. (Courtesy of the Lakso Company, Leominster,
Pennsylvania.)

dislodge and set particles in motion and create a central vortex in
the liquid. This permits the television and electronic system to
detect underfilled, overfilled, or empty containers. The inspection
area of the container is pre-set. Liquid levels that do not exactly
fit within the upper and lower limits of the inspection area are rejected automatically. If the container has the correct fill volume,
it then "becomes eligible" for the inspection process that detects
the presence of foreign matter.

A "master picture" of the correctly filled container is taken simultaneously with the liquid level pictures. The master is put into
Autoskan's electronic memory, which serves as a standard for subsequent comparative video images of the same container. Sixteen
comparison pictures of the container are taken and compared to the
master picture. Any difference between the master and any of the

subsequent comparative pictures of the single container will result in that container being rejected. Since the Autoskan has the capability of inspecting between 1800 and 4500 containers per hour, the time span for checking the liquid level, taking a master picture, and subsequent comparison pictures is less than one second per container.

The fact that the liquid contents are swirling while the container itself is motionless during the inspection process has a very important implication. The master picture is based on a motionless container. All scratches, printing, or other marks on either the outer or inner surface of the container are part of the master picture. Any difference between the master and any one of the subsequent comparison pictures of the single container, therefore, would be caused only by particulate matter moving within the liquid contents, reflecting light back to the camera.

Louer et al. (48) compared Autoskan's performance against visual inspection for discrimination of "good" and "bad" ampul solutions in terms of particulate contamination. Their results, reproduced in Table 3.7, showed that on the average there was a 93% rejection of control bad ampuls by the machine whereas the percentage for visual inspection was only 54%. With the machine, only 7% of the bad ampuls were passed. The rejection of good ampuls by visual inspection was significantly lower.

TABLE 3.7   Comparison of Visual Inspection vs. Autoskan Automatic Inspection of Ampuls for Particulate Matter

	Visual inspection 50 examinations (avg.)	Machine inspection 10 runs
Ampuls (n = 50) rejected from the control "bad" lot	26.6	42.7 out of 46
% of "bad" lot rejected	53.2	92.8
Ampuls rejected from the control "good" lot	3.16	39.6 out of 752
% of "good" lot rejected	0.42	5.25

Source: Ref. 48.

164 / Particulate Matter Testing

Eisai Ampul Inspection Machine (AIM) System

Like the Autoskan system, the Eisai system uses white light as the source of detection of particles. However, whereas Autoskan measures light scattered from a particle, Eisai detects the moving shadows produced by foreign matter in a container of solution. As with the Autoskan, each container is spun around and stopped so that only the liquid in the container is still rotating when the container enters the light. If any foreign matter is floating and rotating in the liquid, the light transmitted through the liquid is blocked and a shadow is cast by the moving particles. Eisai systems employ a phototransistor that converts moving shadows into electrical signals. These signals are compared to pre-set detection sensitivity signal standards and if the standard sensitivity is exceeded, the container is rejected. Like the Autoskan, the Eisai detector does not react to scratches, stains, colors of the ampul or the color of the liquid contents since these are all perceived as stationary objects.

The Eisai system, like the Autoskan system, checks the volume of liquid in the container and can reject overfilled, underfilled, and empty containers. The shadow cast by the liquid meniscus of a properly filled container is expected to fall within a certain preset range within the inspection field. If it falls above or below this range the container is rejected. Adjustments in the Eisai system can be easily made for different ampul sizes, ampul color, and viscosity of the liquid contents.

The conveyance and inspectional mechanism of the Eisai system is shown in Figure 3.3. Ampuls are conveyed by the star wheel onto the inspection table, spun at a high speed, and stopped before reaching the light beam. When the ampul enters the light beam, the light projector and detector follow the ampul while liquid is still rotating inside. After one ampul is inspected by two sets of projectors and receptors (thus, a double inspection system) the next ampul is carried through the same process. Ampuls are moved on by the screw conveyor to the sorting pendulum, where rejected and accepted ampuls are separated. The AIM system automatically keeps count of the number of accepted and rejected containers and displays these numbers on the display panel.

Performance evaluations of the Eisai AIM system have been conducted by at least three major pharmaceutical companies: Upjohn, Organon, and Merck Sharp & Dohme. The complete report of these evaluations is available from Eisai U.S.A., Inc. One evaluation was reported at the 1982 Annual Meeting of the Parenteral Drug Association. All three investigations concluded that the inspection of ampuls by the AIM system compared to manual inspection resulted

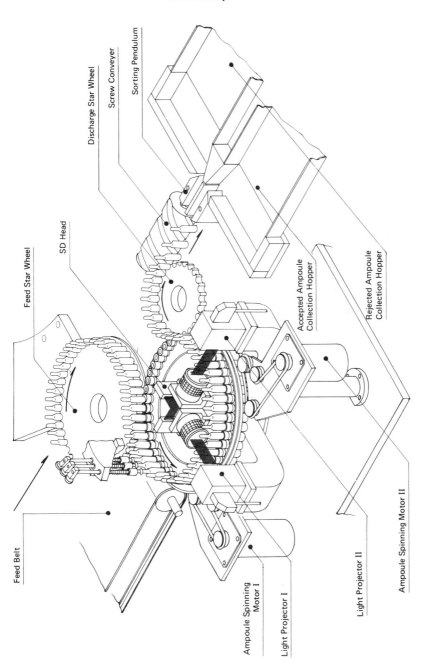

FIGURE 3.3 Conveyance and inspection mechanism of the Eisai automatic inspection system. (Courtesy of Eisai, USA, Inc., Torrance, California.)

in a greater improvement in the quality of ampuls accepted and released. Using the performance criteria model published by J. Knapp et al. (to be discussed in the section "Probabilistic Particulate Detection Model"), Upjohn found that the Eisai machine will do a better job than manual inspection in rejecting defective ampuls for production lots. Organon found the Eisai machine to be more reproducible than human inspection as long as the product in the containers was not an oil or had the tendency to foam. Merck found that the quality of the Eisai inspected material was more than twice the quality of those containers manually inspected. Advantages of the Eisai system itemized by the Merck report include (a) versatility, i.e., ability to handle a large variety of ampul and vial sizes, products, and viscosities, (b) the adjustable sensitivity level, (c) attainable speeds, (d) results of the performance studies, and (e) the price.

   To this author's knowledge, there is no published report directly comparing the inspection performances of Autoskan and Eisai.

Schering PDS/A-V System

Schering Corporation has patented the PDS/A-V, a fully automated particulate inspection system (49). A photograph of the system is shown in Figure 3.4.

   Containers are conveyor-fed from oriented trays into the inspection star wheel. Light is directed into a container using fused fiber optic papes formed into a narrow slit. The container is spun, creating motion of particles in the liquid inside. The entire container is scanned by a fiber optic image dissector, which forms multiple-image planes of the entire liquid volume. The image dissector transmits light scattered from moving particles in the container to a set of matched photodiodes, where the light is changed into an electrical signal and processed. Only signals from moving particles are processed; thus, container defects or printing do not generate false rejects. The image dissector inspects first the lighted lower part of the container for glass particles, then the full volume of the container for other particles, including those floating at the meniscus. Containers are rejected by a single-board microcomputer if the scattered light detected results in a higher score than the digital rejection criteria stored in the computer. The device can inspect 10,000 containers per hour. More elaborate details of the successful automated inspection device are given in the papers published by Knapp et al. (49–53).

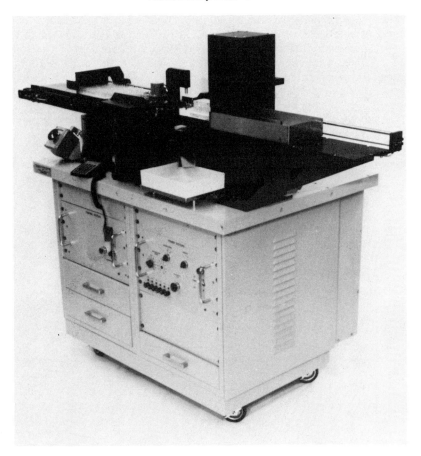

FIGURE 3.4   Particulate Detection System 100 for ampuls and vials.
(Courtesy of Electro-Nucleonics, Inc., Fairfield, New Jersey.)

Probabilistic Particulate Detection Model

Knapp and his co-workers published a series of papers describing
the theory and application of a probabilistic inspection model in
the automated non-destructive particulate analysis of sealed parenteral containers. The probabilistic model is based on the finding
that particulate inspection methodologies, human or robotic, are
probabilistic rather than deterministic in nature (50). In other
words, no final container of solution is acceptable or unacceptable;

rather, each final container of solution possesses a probability of being rejected for whatever inspection process is being evaluated. Rejection probabilities are determined simply by recording the number of times a numbered container is passed and the number of times that same container is rejected during a manual or automatic inspection process. Each container accumulates an accept/reject record. If 1000 containers are inspected several times and each of the 1000 containers yields an accept/reject ratio, a histogram can be constructed plotting the number of containers in each probability group against an empirically determined rejection probability. Such a histogram is shown in Figure 3.5 and represents the corner-

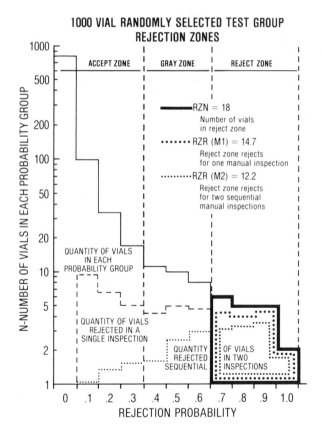

FIGURE 3.5 Histogram plotting number of vials per each probability of rejection group. (Courtesy of J. Z. Knapp, Schering Corporation, Kenilworth, New Jersey.)

stone for the conversion by Knapp et al. of particulate inspection from a craft to a science (53).

The abscissa in Figure 3.5 represents rejection probabilities grouped arbitrarily into 11 intervals. The ordinate represents the logarithmic number of containers (vials) within each of the 11 probability groups. For example, of the 1000 vials inspected for particulate contamination, 805 vials were found to be particulate-free in each of the 50 inspections while 2 vials contained particulates that were detected in each of the 50 inspections.

The dashed lines on the lower half of the histogram show the average number of vials rejected in a single inspection or two sequential inspections in each probability group. These values are obtained from the relationship (50)

$$P (Mn)i = P (Ml)i$$

where $P (Mn)i$ is the rejection probability associated with the nth manual inspection in a probability group, $P (Ml)i$ is the quantity of vials rejected in a rejection probability group in a single inspection, and n is the number of inspections of rejected material. For example, of the eight vials located in the 0.6 rejection probability ($P Ml)i$ group, five were rejected following a single inspection while only three were rejected following two sequential inspections. This indicates that improved discrimination occurs following a reinspection of initial rejects. The reinspection was utilized as a practical response to the existence of particulates even in well-controlled parenteral manufacturing areas below the range of present medical and FDA interest (51). From the information contained in the reinspection histogram of Figure 3.5, Knapp and Kushner (50) defined three zones within the rejection probability limits of 0 and 1.

The accept zone contains all vials that have less than one chance in 10 of rejection in two sequential inspections. The reject zone contains all vials that have at least one chance in two of being rejected in two sequential inspections. The gray zone exists between the accept and reject zones. For single inspections, the probability limits for the three zones are seen in Figure 3.5 where

Accept Zone $\quad p \leqslant 0.3$
Gray Zone $\quad 0.3 \leqslant p \geqslant 0.7$
Reject Zone $\quad p \geqslant 0.7$

Figure 3.5 also shows three terms abbreviated RZN, RZR (M1), and RZR (M2). The definitions of these terms are given in the figure. Their calculations are explained thoroughly in Reference 50.

Using these terms a variety of parameters can be measured, including reject zone efficiency (RZE) and undesired reject rate (RAG). By definition, RZE = RZR/RZN. In the example in Figure 3.5, the RZE after a single inspection is 81.7%. This means an 81.7% probability exists for a manual single inspection method to reject those vials known to exist in the reject zone. Matching or exceeding this objective measure of the security achieved by a manual parenteral inspection procedure should be the only GMP requirement for validation of any alternative inspection technique or process (50).

The availability of the probabilistic model for particle inspection of sterile product solutions in their containers has permitted objective evaluations of various inspection parameters, new methodologies, and new detection equipment. For example, the Schering Particulate Detection System for ampuls (PDS/A) was validated using the probabilistic methodology (49, 51). RZE scores were used to determine the effects of lighting levels, light polarization, and lens magnification on a human inspection of vials mechanically positioned by an experimental machine at Upjohn (54). RZE scores permitted the selection of optimal settings for light, magnification, and light polarization. Interestingly, however, RZE scores also showed that the mechanical handler was not as efficient in meeting the minimum Upjohn standards for performance as their currently used inspection process. The probabilistic model allowed a valid decision to be made based on objective scientific data.

USP TEST FOR PARTICULATE MATTER IN LARGE-VOLUME INJECTIONS FOR SINGLE-DOSE INFUSION

After several years of collaborative effort among laboratories from the FDA, universities, and pharmaceutical manufacturers, a method became official in the First Supplement of the USP (19th edition) in 1975 for the particulate matter analysis and release specifications for single dose large-volume parenterals (LVP). The method involves the filtration of 25 mls of solution through an ultraclean membrane filtration assembly, then observing the membrane and counting entrapped particles on its surface under a microscope using 100× magnification. Analysis by microscopic techniques suffers from several disadvantages—it is very time-consuming, requires technical expertise, and, because of the manpower requirements, can be very expensive. Several alternatives to the approved USP method have been accepted for particle counting, most recently the HIAC electronic particle counter. However, if any disputes arise regarding fulfillment of USP particulate matter specifications, such disputes must be settled by applying the official USP microscopic method.

General

The present USP method provides both qualitative and quantitative data on particulate content in LVP solutions. Particles not less than 10 μm can be counted, sized, and described in terms of their shape and, at times, their nature, e.g., a cotton fiber, piece of glass, or metal sliver. Photographs of the filter membrane further provide a permanent record of the particulate matter test results.

Considerable care and skill are required for preparing the membrane, cleaning the glassware and equipment used in the procedure, and using the microscope. This presents a major disadvantage and motivates pharmaceutical manufacturers to develop and validate alternative methods employing automation, electronic counting instrumentation, or both.

Procedure

Laminar Air Flow (LAF) Hood

All operations and manipulations must be performed under a certified laminar flow hood equipped with ultra HEPA (high efficiency particulate absolute) filters. Air flow velocity must range between 70 and 110 feet per minute as measured with a calibrated velometer. Laminar flow hood certification has been discussed in Chapter 1.

Working in a laminar air flow environment can never replace the necessity for rigid clean technique in sample preparation and analysis. Prior to conducting a test, the hood must be cleaned with an appropriate solvent, preferably 70% ethanol. The HEPA filter itself is not cleaned because of potential damage to the filter surface.

The hood should have a built-in sink or some accommodation for collection and disposal of solvents used in the filtration process.

Introduction and Use of Equipment in the LAF Hood

The USP demands the use of "scrupulously" clean glassware and equipment for the particle test. The word "scrupulous" means the following:

1. Rinse glassware and equipment successively with (a) warm detergent solution, (b) hot water, (c) water, and (d) isopropyl alcohol. The first supplement of the 19th edition of

the USP listed a fifth rinse with trichlorofluoroethane (Freon 113). Freon was eliminated in the 20th edition procedure because of concern about its toxicity in a closed environment.
2. Rinsing technique is important. Glassware and equipment must be rinsed starting at the top of the vertically held object and working downward in a back-and-forth manner. Water rinsing may be done outside the LAF hood, but the final isopropyl alcohol rinse must be performed within the hood.
3. After rinsing, all objects must dry under the hood upstream of all other operations. This helps to ensure that few, if any, extraneous particles adhere to the drying object.

Rubber Gloves

The USP requires the use of suitable, non-powdered gloves for the particle test. Gloves are important in protecting the hands from the dehydrating effects of isopropyl alcohol. However, gloves may create more problems than they solve. Using gloves of improper size will promote problems in careful handling of glassware and equipment. Gloves also produce a false sense of security resulting in less than ideally careful manipulations in the LAF hood. The greatest potential limitation of gloves is the contribution they can make to particulate contamination, even after adequate rinsing. Thus, this requirement continues to be controversial.

Membrane Filter and Assembly

Membranes

The USP specifies that a color contrast grid membrane filter be used, but does not specify the porosity of the membrane. The porosity must be sufficiently small to entrap all particles $\geqslant 10$ μm. Most laboratories use cellulosic type membranes in the porosity range of $0.8-1.2$ μm.

Explicit instructions are provided in the USP for rinsing the membrane filter. In the 19th edition of the USP, Freon was used as the rinsing agent. In the 20th edition, water replaced Freon. Rinsing of a vertically held filter (using forceps) is accomplished using filtered water sprayed from a pressurized container. Rinsing of the membrane with filtered water starts at the top of the non-gridded side, sweeping a stream of water back and forth across the membrane surface from top to bottom. This process is repeated on the gridded side of the membrane. Pressures exceeding 2 psi may damage the delicate membrane.

The rinsing solvent is checked for particle counts, serving as the blank determination in the testing portion of the USP procedure. It must be assumed that no dispensing vessel will provide a particle-free solvent. While the membrane filter on the nozzle will effectively remove particles above the rated porosity of the filter (usually 1.2 µm), particles on the downstream side of the filter on the nozzle will shed into the dispensed solvent. Of course, there is always the possibility of a misplaced or torn membrane filter on the dispenser nozzle.

Filter Assembly

The appropriately rinsed membrane filter is placed with the grid side up on the filter holder base. Great care is taken when the filtering funnel is situated on the base so that the membrane is not rumpled or torn. Prior to placing this assembly on the filtering flask, the unit is rinsed throughly and carefully with filtered water from the pressurized solvent dispenser. After allowing time for the rinse fluid to drain the filter, the apparatus is then secured on top of the filter flask.

Test Preparation

Containers to be tested for particulate matter must be inverted 20 times before the contents are sampled. Agitation has been shown to affect particle size distribution (55) so the 20-fold inversion procedure must be consistent. After rinsing the outer surface of the container with filtered water, the closure is removed. One can never be certain that removal of the closure will not introduce extraneous particles. Careful aseptic and clean technique must be adhered to as much as possible.

After the closure has been carefully removed, the contents are swirled before 25 mls are transferred to the filtering funnel. After standing for one minute, a vacuum is applied to filter the 25 ml sample. Filtered water is then applied with the vacuum off to rinse the walls of the funnel. The stream of filtered water should not hit the filter membrane for fear of tearing the membrane. The rinse fluid then is filtered via vacuum. Unfortunately, particles tend to adhere to the underside of the filter assembly top and to the O rings used between the filter base and filter funnel.

The funnel section of the assembly is carefully removed. The membrane is lifted away from the base using forceps and placed on a plastic Petri slide containing a small amount of stopcock grease or double-sided adhesive tape. The cover of the Petri slide is placed slightly ajar atop the slide to facilitate the membrane drying process. The slide then is placed on the micrometer stage of the microscope for visual analysis.

Particle Count Determination

Examination of the entire membrane filter surface for particulates may be accomplished using a precisely aligned and calibrated microscope. The microscope should be binocular, fitted with a 10 × objective, and have one ocular equipped with a micrometer able to measure accurately particles of 10 µm and 25 µm linear dimension. Incident light should be set at an angle of 10 to 20 degrees, although an angle of 30 to 35 degrees has been reported to be more effective in illuminating the membrane surface inside a plastic Petri slide (56). Calibration of microscope micrometers based on a National Bureau of Standards primary standard stage micrometer has been described by Lanier et al. (57).

Particles are counted under 100 × magnification with the incident light at an angle of 10 to 20 degrees. Obviously, this is a slow and tedious process requiring patience and dedication on the part of the microscopist. Use of higher magnification, up to 400 ×, may be necessary occasionally to discern discrete particles from agglomerates or amorphous masses (56). Sometimes particles not visible with dark field reflected light are very easily observed by means of bright field illumination at 45° polarization.

Two sizes of particles are counted, those having effective linear dimensions ≥10 µm and ≥25 µm. The counts obtained from the sample membranes are compared to counts obtained from a membrane treated exactly like the sample membrane minus the filtration of the product sample. Counts from the "blank" membrane are subtracted from the sample membrane counts. Blank membrane counts rarely are zero. However, if 5 or more particles ≥25 µm are counted on the blank membrane, the test is invalidated and it signifies a serious problem in one or more of the following areas: poor technique, filter breakdown in the solvent dispenser, poorly cleaned membranes, poorly cleaned filter assemblies, and/or HEPA filter leaks. The problem must be resolved before particle testing can resume.

The USP specifically requires all test preparations and blanks to be performed in duplicate. Following the subtraction of blank counts from sample counts and averaging the results, should the net particle counts exceed the limits specified by the USP (not more than 50 particles per ml ≥10 µm and not more than 5 particles per ml ≥25 µm) the large-volume injection product fails the USP test for particulate matter.

PARTICULATE MATTER IN SMALL-VOLUME PARENTERALS

It has been generally accepted that the particle load in large-volume parenteral (LVP) solutions has been substantially reduced because of the USP particle limits placed on these solutions back in 1975 (25). It has also been a general consensus that these LVP limits are too strict for small-volume parenteral (SVP) solutions and, in fact, SVPs should not have particle limits because (a) volumes administered are much smaller than those for LVPs, and (b) health hazards from injected particulates have not been unequivocally established. Nevertheless, the USP over the past several years has conducted studies to establish particle limits for SVP solutions that are reasonable from both a safety standpoint and a quality control standpoint achievable by the parenteral industry.

Two SVP particle limit proposals were published in late 1983 (58). One based on particles per container was proposed by the USP Subcommittee on Parenteral Products; the other proposal, by the USP Panel on Sterile Products, was based on particles per ml. A comparison of the two proposals is summarized below:

	>25 μm	>10 μm
Subcommittee proposal	1000 Particles per container	10,000 Particles per container
Panel on Sterile Products proposal	70 Particles per ml	250 Particles per ml

The subcommittee proposed limits based on the following rationale: the addition of up to five containers of any SVP to a 1 liter LVP solution should not increase the number of particles by more than double those allowed by the USP limit for LVP solutions (five particles per ml >25 μm or 5000 particles in 1 liter >25 μm; 50 particles per ml >10 μm or 50,000 particles in 1 liter >10 μm). If five additives, each containing no more than 1000 particles per container >25 μm, were admixed with the 1 liter LVP containing 5000 particles >25 μm, the total particles >25 μm would be 10,000, which would be the maximum allowable particle number per admixed solution. At 10 μm, the total particle number with five additives in a 1 liter LVP would be 100,000, which would be no more than double that of the LVP alone. Therefore the subcommittee proposal is based upon concern more for the cumulative particulate insult the patient receives than for the number of particles per ml of solution.

The USP panel proposal was based on data from an FDA survey of a large number of small-volume parenterals. Particle counts were obtained from an electronic particle counter (HIAC). After combining data from all the samples (157 samples of 19 aqueous drug products, 10 units per each sample), the upper 95% confidence limits of the means at 25 μm and at 10 μm were those listed above.

Of the more than 500 official SVP products in the USP, 134 of these products (58) meet the following criteria for selection of products subject to particulate matter limit:

1. The drug is usually administered via the artery or vein, or intrathecally.
2. The drug is likely to be used continuously or repeatedly for a course of treatment.
3. Drugs solely for emergency use for diagnostic procedures, for anti-cancer therapy, or for episodic use are excluded.

While many laboratories prefer to employ the LVP microscopic method for counting particles in SVP products, the USP XXI introduced the use of an electronic liquid-borne particle counter system. Initial controversy over the test resulted in a postponement of the test becoming official until July, 1985. The major complaint of the new USP method centered around the use of the HIAC-Royko electronic particle counter (see page 181). Like any electronic counting device, the HIAC cannot identify and characterize particles, cannot accurately measure a particle's longest dimension (i.e. measures all particles as spheres), will count silicon and air bubbles as particles and standardization/ calibration of the HIAC can be difficult. Also, many manufacturers objected to being forced to use an instrument which is available from only one major U.S. supplier.

Other concerns over the proposed USP test for SVP particulate matter included lack of a sufficient data base from which limits were established, lack of validation of the USP proposed method, the basis for requiring particle limits for some products but not for others in individual monographs, problems in specific details in the calibration, preparation and determination sections of the test, and the lack of consistency between the LVP and SVP tests for particulate matter.

AUTOMATED USP PARTICULATE MATTER TEST

Human variables unavoidably decrease the accuracy, precision, and reproducibility of manually measuring particulate matter using the USP microscopic method. As pointed out by Clements and Swenson (59), considerable time and concentration are required even under ideal circumstances for the microscopist to perform the necessary operations to obtain a clear and accurate view of a particle's longest dimension. Viewing multiple particles adds to the complexity of time and concentration. Parallax errors (differences in sizing a particle when seen from two different points not on a straight line with the particle) decrease accuracy, especially when measuring smaller (e.g., 5—10 µm) particles. In summary, the success of application of the manual microscopic technique is directly proportional to the microscopist's efficiency, which, in turn, is dependent upon his or her speed, concentration, and alertness.

To minimize or eliminate the human factor in the USP particulate matter test, a number of electronic particle-counting instruments have been developed, refined, and computerized for rapid and relatively accurate and reproducible particle measurements. However, the main disadvantage of electronic particle counting from a regulatory point of view is a lack of adherence to the official USP test. As previously noted, electronic instrumentation for particle counting is permitted to satisfy USP particle test requirements for large-volume injectables. However, in cases of controversy, the USP microscopic method must be the final judge.

The nearest equivalent automated system to the USP manual microscopic method is a system called image analysis. The system described here differs from the automated inspection systems that were described in the section "Visual Inspection: Automatic Methods." Image analysis is not a 100% final container inspection system. Rather, this system introduces automation after the large-volume parenteral sample has been filtered and the membrane prepared. Particle analysis of the filter membrane is performed by a computer-controlled microscope and television system.

The Quantimet automated image analysis system has been fully explained in the literature (59). According to USP procedure, the membrane filter, following filtration, is mounted in a plastic filter holder and placed securely on the microscope stage plate. An external fiber optic illuminator provides low-angle, high-intensity illumination with directional control to satisfy USP requirements and to create optimum particle contrast against the filter background. Optically interfaced to the microscope is a high-resolution television camera. Each field of the filter surface imaged by the microscope is scanned by the camera, which produces a digital picture containing geometric and densitometric information. The camera signal is processed by the central processor, where data representing the longest dimension of each particle on the filter surface are fed to the output computer for processing and presentation. Results can be displayed on the video monitor, printed to provide a permanent hard copy record, and stored on magnetic discs for future recall. To meet USP requirements, data generally are reported as the number of particles having effective linear dimensions equal to or greater than 10 μm and equal to or greater than 25 μm.

Millipore Corporation developed a particle-measurement computer system similar in theory, instrumentation, and application to the Quantimet system (60). The πMC system consists of (a) a microscope and television camera that illuminate and observe the sample on the filter membrane, (b) a computer module that receives the video signals from the television camera and applies the appropriate logic to count and measure particles in the viewing area, and (c) a viewing monitor that subsequently receives the video signal, reconstructs the field of view, and prints the desired particle data at the top of the monitoring screen.

The advantages of automated microscopic analytical systems in review are:

1. They conform to USP procedure for particle analysis of large-volume injectable solutions.
2. Particles are counted, sized, and shape-characterized with much greater speed and precision as compared with the manual microscopic method.
3. Efficiency and reproducibility are increased while tedium is eliminated.
4. Permanent records in the form of particle data and photomicrographs can be obtained.
5. Operation of these systems requires minimal technical and manipulative skills.

ELECTRONIC PARTICLE COUNTERS

The limitations of human inspection and microscopic analytical methods in the detection of particulate matter in injectable products have already been addressed. While not officially recognized in compendial literature as of January, 1985, electronic particle-counting methods have been applied in the parenteral industry in a variety of ways (see Table 3.8).

Two major advantages of electronic particle counters are their automated characteristics and the rapidity at which they do particulate analysis. Three major disadvantages hinder electronic

TABLE 3.8   Application of Electronic
Particle Counters in the Parenteral Industry

---

1. Small-volume parenterals
2. Large-volume parenterals
3. Deionized water, water for injection, USP
4. Rubber closures
5. Hypodermic syringes
6. Administration sets

---

particle analysis from becoming a more acceptable means of measuring for particulate contamination: electronic particle counters are
expensive; they cannot differentiate among various types of particles; and they measure particle size differently from microscopic
analysis. Comparisons of the various methods of detecting particles in parenteral solutions will be discussed in the section "Comparison of Microscopic and Electronic Particle-Counting Methods."
A practical understanding of the operational principles of the three
types of electronic liquid particle counters is essential before one
can competently compare one particle counting method to another.

Principle of Electrical Resistivity (Coulter Counter) (61—63)

The Coulter Counter (Figure 3.6) detects particles by measuring
the change in electrical resistance produced when a particle dis-
places a part of the electrolyte solution residing between two electrodes. The change in resistance is directly proportional to the
volume of the particle (64). The Coulter Counter, therefore, treats
a particle as a three-dimensional object. This can be contrasted to
the light-blockage principle, which views a particle in two dimensions and, thus, calculates area rather than volume of a particle.
     Coulter Counters employ an aperture tube with a known micron
opening that is immersed in a volume of parenteral solution. The
ratio of particle diameter to orifice diameter should be less than 0.3
for the direct proportionality of resistance change and particle
volume to be valid (64). For example, a 50 μm or greater aperture
tube should be used for counting particles in the 10 μm size range.
     Particle analysis must take place in a controlled clean room under
HEPA-filtered air to minimize environmental particles entering the
sample solution. The aperture tube is immersed in the intravenous
solution, which must be electrolytic. If not, an electrolyte solution
(e.g., sterile sodium chloride for injection) must be added. This

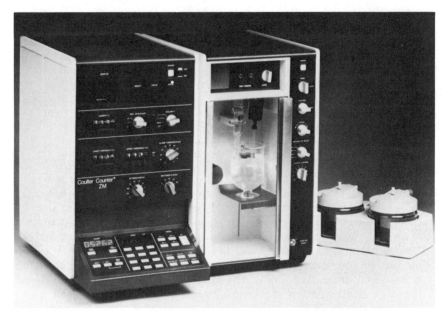

FIGURE 3.6   Photograph of Coulter Counter Model ZM.   (Courtesy of Coulter Electronics, Inc., Hialeah, Florida.)

presents a major disadvantage in the use of the Coulter Counter if an electrolytic solution must be added. The solution itself may add a significant number of particles to the sample solution. Appropriate blank controls must be utilized to subtract the particulate contribution caused by the added electrolytic solution.

The instrument employs a manometer to sample from 500 µl to 2 ml of the I.V. solution. Counts measured in this extremely small volume may be too low (10—20 particles) for useful statistical accuracy of sampling (65). Air bubbles adversely affect accurate counting. Air bubbles are avoided by either minimized agitation during sampling or application of a vacuum before measurement. Electrical background noise also contributes to some error in actual counting of submicronic particles.

Sample solution is pulled through the aperture of the Coulter Counter solution tube and flows between two electrodes. The change in resistance, proportional to particle volume, creates a signal that is relayed to a threshold analyzer. The threshold analyzer has been previously calibrated so that only pulses of voltage exceeding the threshold position are counted. The pulses generated are displayed on an oscilloscope by electronic amplification. Voltage pulse heights are proportional to the amplifier gain and aperature current of the instrument and the resistance changes due to the passage of the particles (3).

The signal produced is proportional to the volume of electrolyte solution displaced by the particle. The count display is a function of volume directly or the diameter of a sphere of equal volume (66). The Coulter Counter can count up to 5000 particles per second using the Coulter principle of one-by-one counting and sizing. Size distributions can be accurately determined over a range of 0.5 to 800 μm, depending on the proper selection of optimal glassware.

Particulate matter in the subvisible size range present in intravenous solutions can be detected easily and rapidly by the Coulter Counter (65, 67–71). Because of its electrical resistivity principle, the Coulter Counter especially applies in the determination of particulate contamination in parenteral electrolyte solutions such as those containing sodium chloride. Coulter Counters obtain particle size data with no indication regarding the shape or composition of the particles. The diameter of particles measured by the Coulter Counter is a mean spherical diameter. Since particles found in I.V. solutions are usually not spherical, it is important for the orifice dimension of the Coulter aperture tube to be much greater than the size of particles monitored by the counter. Acicular particles having lengths much smaller than the diameter of the aperture orifice will produce more accurate pulse heights having magnitudes closely corresponding to the total volume of the particle.

Principle of Light Blockage (HIAC)

A schematic representation of the light-blockage principle is shown in Figure 3.7. A tungsten lamp produces a constant collimated beam of light which passes through a small rectangular passageway and impinges onto a photodiode. In a clear passageway the light intensity received by the photodiode remains constant.

Liquids can flow through the passageway between the light source and the photodiode. If a single particle transverses the light beam, there results a reduction in the normal amount of light received by the photodiode. This reduction of light and the measurable decrease in the output from the photodiode is proportional to the area of the particle interrupting the light flow. Thus, the light-blockage principle measures particle size based on the diameter of a circle having an equivalent area.

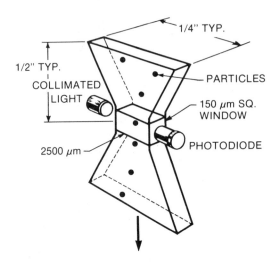

FIGURE 3.7   Schematic representation of the light blockage principle. (Courtesy of HIAC/Royko, Menlo Park, California.)

HIAC (High Accuracy Instruments Division) particle counters employ the light-blockage principle in the detection and quantitation of particulate matter in parenteral solutions (see Figure 3.8). These instruments count approximately 4000 particles per second. HIAC counters use sensors having size measurement ratios of 1:60. In other words, a 1 through 60 micrometer sensor can measure particles from 1 to 60 μm, while a 2.5 through 150 micrometer sensor can measure particles ranging from 2.5 to 150 μm. Channel numbers on the counter are selected and calibrated according to the size range desired.

Increasingly, over the past several years, HIAC systems have progressed in technological advances and user application in the particle analysis field. Advantages for using HIAC particle counters have outweighed the disadvantages. Lantz et al. (72) were among the first to publish results of HIAC analyses of parenteral solution particulate contamination. In conclusion, the advantages and disadvantages of using the HIAC particle counter were as follows:

Advantages

1. Particles are counted automatically.
2. Parenteral solutions, either electrolytes or non-electrolytes, could be counted.

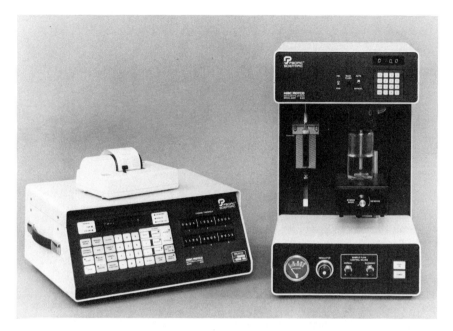

FIGURE 3.8   Models 3000 and 4100 HIAC/Royko Particle Counter. (Courtesy of HIAC/Royko, Menlo Park, California.)

3. The instrument was easy to calibrate and use.
4. Replication of counts was good.
5. Ability to vary the volume of sample as desired for counting.
6. Dilution method of counting permitted counting of both "clean" and heavily contaminated solution.
7. Direct method of counting permitted counting of crystallized soluble particles.

Disadvantages

1. Instrument is relatively expensive as compared to equipment used for counting by optical microscope.
2. Particulate contaminants cannot be identified.
3. Large and/or fibrous particles may block the sensor opening.
4. Air bubbles are counted as particulate matter.
5. Dilution method of counting does not permit counting of crystallized soluble materials because dilution solubilizes crystals.

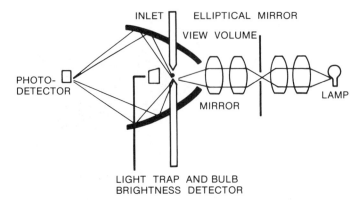

FIGURE 3.9   Schematic representation of the light-scattering principle.   (Courtesy of Climet Instruments Co., Redlands, California.)

Principle of Light Scattering

When a beam of light strikes a solid object, three events occur: some of the light is absorbed; some of the light is transmitted; and the rest of the light is scattered. Scattered light is a composite of diffracted, refracted, and reflected light. Particle counters that operate on the basis of light scattering are designed to measure the intensity of light scattered at fixed angles to the direction of the light beam. A schematic example is given in Figure 3.9.

As a liquid flows into a light sensing zone, particles in the fluid scatter light in all directions. The scattered light is directed onto a system of elliptical mirrors which then focus the light onto a photodetector. The light trap seen in Figure 3.9 is designed to absorb most of the main light beam photons.

The Royko and Climet particle counters represent examples of counters operating under this principle. Davies and Smart (73) reported on rapid assessment of particle levels in small-volume ampul products with good reproducibility using the Royko. Advantages and disadvantages of the Royko counter and other counters based on light scattering are similar to those identified for the HIAC counter described above.

COMPARISON OF MICROSCOPIC AND ELECTRONIC PARTICLE-COUNTING METHODS

The comparisons discussed in this section will include methods capable of quantitating particulate contamination, i.e., microscopic and electronic methods. Comparisons involving visual inspection, both manual and automated methods, were discussed in the section "Comparison to Other Particle Inspection Methods."

Difficulties in comparing particle-counting methods result from differences in the way in which different methods determine particle size and distribution. For example, the microscopic method measures size as the longest linear dimension of the particle. The principle of light blockage, utilized by the HIAC particle counter, expresses size as the diameter of a circle of equivalent area as the actual area consumed by the particle. Particle counting by electrical resistance (Coulter Counter) treats the particle as a three-dimensional object and measures the volume consumed by the particle. Thus, the microscope, HIAC, and Coulter Counter methods size particles in one, two, and three dimensions, respectively.

An excellent theoretical discussion by Schroeder and DeLuca (66) showed that it is virtually impossible to correlate instrumental and microscopic particle counts directly for irregularly shaped particles. As seen in Table 3.9, as long as the particle is a sphere, all methods will size the sphere equally. However, as the particle shape deviates from sphericity, the size measurement by the three alternate approaches will differ, sometimes drastically, from the value obtained by the USP microscopic method. For example, if the solution sample contained 50 ellipsoid particles with their longest linear dimension equaling 10 μm, the HIAC will yield a count of 50 × 0.61 = 30.5 particles. In fact, this HIAC value may be an overestimate because the 0.61 correction factor considers only size (10 μm), not the actual number of particles. Assuming that the size-count relationship follows the conventional log-log relationship, the theoretical HIAC count of 50 ellipsoid particles of 10 μm size would be only 14.4 particles. Figure 3.10 provides the explanation. The USP microscopic method follows a log-log distribution, yielding a straight-line slope between 10 μm and 25 μm for its pass/fail criteria of 50 particles/ml at 10 μm and 5 particles/ml at 25 μm. Assuming the HIAC method to follow the same log-log distribution between 10 μm and 25 μm, its slope will be parallel to the USP slope. However, the HIAC correlation factor for ellipsoid particles theoretically is 0.61 that of the USP method. Thus, the starting point for the HIAC method is not 10 μm but 6.1 μm at the 50 count position on the log-log graph. Therefore, following a parallel relationship with the slope of the USP method, the HIAC method yields a theoretical particle count value of 14.4 particles at the point intersecting the vertical line from the particle size of 10 μm.

This same logic can be assumed for the Coulter Counter method. From Table 3.10, the size correction factor of the Coulter Counter

TABLE 3.9   Summary of Sphericity Correction Factors Based on Longest Linear Dimension

Shape	D_O Longest dimension	D_H Horizontal projection	D_A Light blockage	D_V Electrolyte displacement
Sphere	1.00	1.00	1.00	1.00
Cube (1:1:1)	1.00	0.90	0.95	0.88
Equant (3:2:1)	1.00	0.88	0.81	0.62
Prolate ellipsoid (2:7:1)	1.00	0.87	0.61	0.52
Flake (4:4:1)	1.00	0.90	0.81	0.55
Rod (3:1 dia.)	1.00	0.81	0.62	0.52
Fiber (rigid, 10:1)	1.00	0.64	0.36	0.25

Source: Ref. 66.

for ellipsoid-shaped particles is 0.52. Applying the same log-log relationship for a 50 particle/ml sample, the Coulter Counter will yield a count of only 9.7 particles of size 10 µm or larger.

Hopkins and Young (74) were the first investigators to publish actual particle size and number data from typical parenteral solutions analyzed by the microscope, HIAC, and Coulter Counter methods. Some of their results are reproduced in Tables 3.11 and 3.12. Table 3.11 shows that the Coulter Counter yielded particle counts that deviated between +9.2 and +40.8% from counts obtained with the microscope. The HIAC counts were between −19.2 and +3.8% from those of the microscope. Table 3.12 demonstrates that (a) the agreement among the three methods was acceptable, especially considering their different mechanisms of particle sizing and the fact that these data all fell well within the Australian particle standard (100 particles/ml ≥5 µm) present at that time (USP standard was not official at that time), and (b) great error is produced in

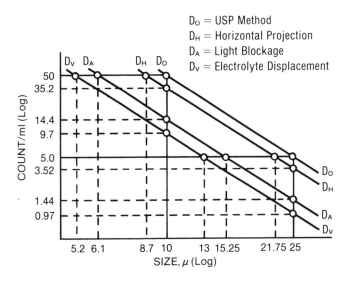

FIGURE 3.10   Log count vs. log size corrections for sizing and counting prolate ellipsoids.   (From Ref. 66.)

TABLE 3.10   Count Comparison Between USP and Electrolyte Displacement Methods

Shape	USP count	SCF	Displacement count at	
			10 μm	6.6 μm
Sphere	5	1.00	5.00	14.20
Cube	5	0.88	3.63	10.30
Equant	15	0.62	4.51	12.82
Ellipsoid	10	0.52	1.93	5.49
Flake	5	0.55	1.11	3.16
Rod	5	0.52	0.97	2.75
Fiber	5	0.25	0.15	0.44
Total/ml	50		17.30	49.16

Source: Ref. 66.

TABLE 3.11   Comparison of Microscope, Coulter, and HIAC Data, Showing Total Counts of Particles Greater than 5 μm

Sample	Microscope	Coulter	HIAC
5606A, Supplier A	6,285	6,867	5,080
5606A, Supplier B	19,364	23,534	18,000
5606A, Supplier B	5,113	7,200	5,020
5606A, Supplier A	4,285	4,635	3,660
5606A, Supplier A	6,675	8,715	6,930

Source: Ref. 74.   Data from Technical Documentary Report No. ML-TDR-64-72, Air Force Materials Laboratory, Wright-Patterson Air Force Base, Ohio.

TABLE 3.12   Particles per ml of Isotonic Saline Solutions in the 5–50 μm Size Range

		HIAC	Coulter	Microscope
MFG A S-1[a]	Average	10.8	17.4	11.9
MFG B S-2[a]	Average	19.2	15.1	11.4
MFG B S-3	Average	7.4	9.7	8.6
MFG B S-4		9.9	6.6	7.9
		10.3	9.2	8.1
		8.7	7.4	8.3
	Average	9.6	7.7	8.1
Filtered water blank		0.9		

[a]Air bubbles in solution.
Source: Ref. 74.

TABLE 3.13 Particulate Matter Determination of Some Intravenous Solutions by Automatic and Microscopic Methods

Infusion solutions	Microscopic method[a]		Image analyzer[b]	Automatic[c]	
	I	II		I	II
5% Dextrose	2869 ± 336	2604 ± 180	2936 ± 275	2673 ± 192	1748 ± 172
5% Dextrose + 0.2% NaCl	2003 ± 127	1928 ± 222	2058 ± 159	1813 ± 125	1223 ± 80
5% Dextrose + 0.45% NaCl	1863 ± 67	1708 ± 119	1642 ± 102	1680 ± 89	879 ± 23
Lactated Ringer's solution	2078 ± 304	2009 ± 200	2096 ± 190	2039 ± 156	1032 ± 105
0.9% Sodium chloride	1247 ± 136	1201 ± 99	1205 ± 271	1250 ± 201	705 ± 176
10% Protein hydrolysate	7374 ± 267	7408 ± 231	4509 ± 160	7185 ± 879	4252 ± 507

[a]Reichert Zetopan Universal Microscope. I, Incident polarized light and polycarbonate as substrate; II, incident bright field lighting and cleared white cellulosic substrate.
[b]TIMC computer measurement method with cleared white cellulosic substrates.
[c]HIAC counter, calibrated with I, AC Fine Test Dust, II, polystyrene-divinylbenzene spheres.
Source: Ref. 75.

both Coulter and HIAC assays when no attempt has been made to exclude air bubbles from the sample solutions. These instruments do count air bubbles as particles; thus, vacuum techniques must be applied to eliminate air bubbles before any instrumental particle counting is performed.

A similar conclusion was reached by Rebagay et al. (75) in that an automatic particle counter can be used in place of either a polarizing microscope or an image-analyzing system for routine particulate matter monitoring of various particle systems (AC Test Dust, polystyrene spheres, antibiotic, electrolyte and large-volume parenteral solutions). However, to do this, the particle counter must be carefully calibrated with particles that possess morphological and optical characteristics similar to the particles of interest. An example of their data measuring particle content of various intravenous infusion solutions is given in Table 3.13.

Lim et al. (76) filtered various small-volume parenteral solutions and counted particles using the manual counting method under the microscope and the electronic Millipore MC method. In products with relatively few particles, both methods gave similar results. In products containing a high number of particles in the size range of 5–25 μm, the electronic method detected more particles. These authors concluded that the electronic method was preferable because of its greater rapidity and precision. A somewhat similar conclusion was made by Blanchard et al. (77) in comparing the microscope and the Prototron laser beam (using the light-scattering principle). With solutions containing more abundant particles of the small-sized range, the particle counter gave more reliable and accurate results than did the microscope.

FACTORS AFFECTING ACCURATE PARTICLE TESTING

Nearly every scientific paper featuring the use of a particle test method, be it visual, microscopic, electronic, manual, or automatic, has to alert the reader to one or more major limitations to the method. These limitations have been addressed in this chapter. For example, visual examination by human beings is limited by its tedium and subjectiveness. Microscopes often are improperly calibrated. Electronic particle counters count air bubbles as particles. For LVPs the USP relies on membrane filtration in which particles from the equipment, environment, or personnel involved in conducting the test inadvertently become deposited on the filter.

Other problems exist that can potentially cause inaccurate particle test results regardless of the test used. Ernerot (78) pointed

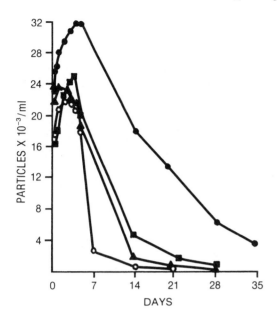

FIGURE 3.11 Number of particles between 2.33 and 5.02 μm found in resting plastic bags after shaking for 30 hours as a function of time and temperature. Key: ■, 35°C; ○, 45°C; ▲, 55°C; ●, room temperature. (From Ref. 79.)

out that the particle contents of injection containers vary considerably between the date of production and a later date when the same containers are tested again. It was found that storage causes particle agglomeration. Mechanical agitation breaks up the agglomerates, resulting in counts that cannot reproduce the original count or replicate one another on the same date of testing. Freshly prepared solutions seemed to give more stable counts. It was suggested that only the manufacturer, who can reproduce the handling of its products, use particle counting as a meaningful control method.

Agitation or shaking will increase the number of particles in a parenteral solution. Blanchard et al. (56) found that the slope and number of particles per milliliter greater than 1 μm in a log-log plot of number against diameter depended on the degree of agitation.

Agitation of LVP by 20 hand inversions, as required by the USP procedure, removed particulate matter from the surface of the container, thus increasing the total number of particles greater than

1 μm. Yet the relative size distribution of particles was not altered significantly. Agitation for 30 minutes disintegrated agglomerates, greatly increased the number of particles with diameters less than 1 μm, and brought about a corresponding decrease in the number of particles exceeding 1 μm in diameter. Particle-counting procedures must be carried out that do not impose a sheer force upon the particles and affect the reproducibility of the test results.

Temperature affects the number of particles found in parenteral solutions. As shown in Figure 3.11 (79), particle number increased as a function of temperature and time. Interestingly and without clear explanation, a decrease in the particle number occurred after 120 hours of storage at all temperatures. Since the particle size range studied was 2.33 to 5.02 μm (using the Coulter Counter), it is possible that particle agglomeration occurred, resulting in a decrease in particle number at these smaller diameters but an increase in particle counts at larger sizes. These same investigators found that glass containers produced fewer particles than plastic containers under similar storage and handling conditions.

REFERENCES

1. United States Pharmacopeia, 21st edition, Mack Publishing, Easton, Pennsylvania, 1985, p. 1137.
2. United States Pharmacopeia, 21st edition, Mack Publishing, Easton, Pennsylvania, 1985, p. 1257.
3. M. J. Groves, *Parenteral Products*, William Heinemann, London, 1973.
4. E. W. Godding, Foreign matter in solutions for injection, *Pharm. J.*, *154*, 124 (1945).
5. United States Pharmacopeia, 13th edition, Mack Publishing, Easton, Pennsylvania, 1947.
6. J. H. Brewer and J. H. F. Dunning, An *in vitro* and *in vivo* study of glass particles in ampuls, *J. Amer. Pharm. Assoc.*, *36*, 289 (1947).
7. N. Leelarasamee, S. A. Howard, and H. J. Baldwin, Visible particle limits in small-volume parenterals, *J. Parenter. Drug Assoc.*, *34*, 167−174 (1980).
8. B. E. Konwaler, Pulmonary emboli of cotton fibers, *Am. J. Clin. Pathol.*, *20*, 385 (1950).
9. W. B. Wartman, B. Hudson, and R. B. Jennings, Experimental arterial disease: The role of the pulmonary artery to emboli of filter paper fibers, *Circul.*, *4*, 756 (1951).

10. E. Gnadinger, A new procedure for the control of injection solutions, thesis, University of Strawbourg, 1957.

11. J. M. Garvan and B. W. Gunner, Intravenous fluids: A solution containing such particles must not be used, *Med. J. Austral.*, *2*, 140 (1963).

12. J. M. Garvan and B. W. Gunner, The harmful effects of particles in intravenous fluids, *Med. J. Austral.*, *2*, 1 (1964).

13. R. M. Geisler, The biological effects of polystyrene latex particles administered intravenously to rats: A collaborative study, *Bull. Parenter. Drug Assoc.*, *27*, 101 (1973).

14. K. Hozumi, K. Kitamura, T. Kitade, and S. Iwagami, Localization of glass particles in animal organs derived from cutting of glass ampoules before intravenous injections, *Microchem. J.*, *28*, 215–226 (1983).

15. J. E. Dimmick, Fiber embolization: A hazard of cardiac surgery and catheterization, *New Engl. J. Med.*, *292*, 685 (1975).

16. P. P. DeLuca, R. R. Rapp, B. Bivins, H. E. McKean, and W. O. Griffin, Filtration and infusion phlebitis: A double-blind prospective clinical study, *Amer. J. Hosp. Pharm.*, *32*, 101 (1975).

17. S. Turco and R. E. King, *Sterile Dosage Forms*, Lea & Febiger, Philadelphia, Pennsylvania, 1979, pp. 411–419.

18. R. J. Duma and M. J. Akers, Parenteral drug administration: Routes, precautions, problems, and complications, *Pharmaceutical Dosage Forms: Parenteral Medications*, (K. E. Avis, L. Lachman, and H. Lieberman, eds.), Marcel Dekker, New York, 1984.

19. P. O. DeLuca, Particulate matter in parenteral products, *Pharm. Tech.*, *3*, 30 (1979).

20. R. G. Draftz and J. Graf, Identifying particle contaminants, *Bull. Parenter. Drug Assoc.*, *28*, 35 (1974).

21. W. C. McCrone, Identification of parenteral particulate contaminants, *Pharm. Tech.*, *2*, 57 (1978).

22. United States Pharmacopoeia, eighth edition, Blakiston, Pennsylvania, 1905.

23. G. Schwartzman, Particulate matter as viewed by the FDA, *Bull. Parenter. Drug Assoc.*, *31*, 161 (1977).

24. National Formulary, sixth edition, Mack Publishing, Easton, Pennsylvania, 1936.

25. First Supplement to United States Pharmacopeia (19th edition) and National Formulary (14th edition), USP Convention, Inc., Rockville, Maryland, 1975, pp. 56–57.

26. I. Vessey and C. E. Kendall, Determination of particulate matter in intravenous fluids, *Analyst, 91*, 273 (1966).

27. *Proposed General Standard for Injections, Particulate Matter in Large-Volume Injections*, National Biological Standards Laboratory, Canberra, Australia, 1974.

28. British Pharmacopoeia, Volume II, Appendix XIII, Her Majesty's Stationery Office, London, England, 1980, p. A120.

29. D. M. Hailey, A. R. Lea, and C. E. Kendall, Specifications of limits for particulate contamination in pharmaceutical dosage forms, *J. Pharm. Pharmacol., 34*, 615—620 (1982).

30. M. J. Groves, Modern techniques for the control of particulate contamination in parenteral solutions, *Cron. Farm., 20*, 212—217 (1977).

31. M. J. Groves and D. Wana, A comparison of instrumental techniques for the determination of contamination in filtered aqueous solutions, *Powder Tech., 18*, 215—223 (1977).

32. W. E. Hamlin, General guidelines for the visual inspection of parenteral products in final containers and in-line inspection of container components, *J. Parenter. Drug. Assoc., 32*, 63 (1978).

33. W. D. Graham, L. G. Chatten, M. Pernarowski, C. E. Cox, and J. M. Airth, A collaborative study on the detection of particles in ampuled solutions, *Drug Standards, 27*, 61 (1959).

34. H. J. Baldwin, S. A. Howard, and N. Leelarasamee, Visual ampul inspection by experienced and non-experienced inspectors, *J. Parenter. Sci. Tech., 35*, 148 (1981).

35. D. Schipper and R. Gaines, Comparison of optical electronic inspection and manual visual inspection, *J. Parenter. Drug Assoc., 32*, 118 (1978).

36. A. C. V. M. Faesen, Reproducibility of visual inspection of parenterals, *J. Parenter. Drug. Assoc., 32*, 75 (1978).

37. P. R. Rasanen and R. C. Louer, Panel discussion: Mechanical inspection of ampuls I—Ampul inspection using Autoskan equipment, *Bull. Parenter. Drug Assoc., 27*, 243 (1973).

38. A. B. McGinn, Panel discussion: Mechanical inspection of ampuls II—Ampul inspection using the Rota machine, *Bull. Parenter. Drug Assoc., 27*, 247 (1973).

39. R. J. Walsh and J. A. Monahan, Panel discussion: Mechanical inspection of ampuls III—Ampul inspection using the Strunck machine, *Bull. Parenter. Drug Assoc., 27*, 250 (1973).

40. J. Blanchard, C. M. Thompson, and J. A. Schwartz, Comparison of methods for detection of particulate matter in

large-volume parenterals, *Amer. J. Hosp. Pharm.*, *33*, 144 (1976).

41. J. B. Wynn, Mechanization of ampoule inspection, *Bull. Parenter. Drug Assoc.*, *22*, 13 (1968).

42. G. W. Martyn, Utilization of Rondo unscrambler and Strunck units in ampoule inspection, *Bull. Parenter. Drug Assoc.*, *24*, 281 (1970).

43. S. Levine, Particulate matter: III. Electronic inspection, *Bull. Parenter. Drug Assoc.*, *20*, 33 (1966).

44. W. E. Hamlin, W. W. Scothorn, and K. W. Riebe, Experience with a prototype television inspection device: I. Detectability of subvisible particles, *Bull. Parenter. Drug Assoc.*, *31*, 86 (1977).

45. B. H. Kaye, Statistical strategies and ROEPA (robot for examining parenterals), *Bull. Parenter. Drug Assoc.*, *33*, 239 (1979).

46. M. J. Groves, Detection of particles in intravenous solution using the nuclepore prototron counter, *Pharm. J.*, *213*, 518 (1974).

47. M. C. Porter, New particle counter for nondestructive monitoring of parenterals, *Pharm. J.*, *29*, 169 (1975).

48. R. C. Louer, J. A. Russoman, and P. R. Rasanen, Detection of particulate matter in parenteral solutions by image projection: A concept and its feasibility, *Bull. Parenter. Drug Assoc.*, *25*, 54 (1971).

49. J. Z. Knapp and H. K. Kushner, Implementation and automation of a particle detection system for parenteral products, *J. Parenter. Drug Assoc.*, *34*, 369 (1980).

50. J. Z. Knapp and H. K. Kushner, Generalized methodology for evaluation of parenteral inspection procedures, *J. Parenter. Drug. Assoc.*, *34*, 14 (1980).

51. J. Z. Knapp, H. K. Kushner, and L. R. Abramson, Automated particulate detection for ampuls with the use of the probabilistic particulate detection model, *J. Parenter. Sci.*, *Tech.*, *35*, 21 (1981).

52. J. Z. Knapp, H. K. Kushner, and L. R. Abramson, Particulate inspection of parenteral products: An assessment, *J. Parenter. Sci.*, *Tech.*, *35*, 176 (1981).

53. J. Z. Knapp and H. K. Kushner, Particulate inspection of parenteral products: From biophysics to automation, *J. Parenter. Sci.*, *Tech.*, *36*, 121 (1982).

54. C. H. Rothrock, R. Gaines, and T. Greer, Evaluating different inspection parameters, *J. Parenter. Sci.*, *Tech.*, *37*, 64 (1983).

55. J. Blanchard, J. A. Schwartz, and D. M. Byrne, Effects of agitation on size distribution of particulate matter in large-volume parenterals, *J. Pharm. Sci.*, *66*, 935 (1977).

56. M. A. Wente, Particulate matter levels in large-volume inspections: USP XIX method, *Bull. Parenter. Drug Assoc.*, *31*, 165 (1977).

57. J. M. Lanier, G. S. Oxborrow, and L. T. Kononen, Calibration of microscopes for measuring particles found in parenteral solutions, *J. Parenter. Drug Assoc.*, *32*, 145 (1978).

58. Particulate matter standards for small-volume injections, *Pharm. Forum*, Nov.–Dec. 1983, 3729–3735.

59. B. Clements and R. Swenson, Automated microscopy for contamination control, *Pharm. Tech.*, *2*, 42 (1978).

60. J. W. Warren, Jr., T. E. Needham, and J. D. Benmaman, Particulate matter detection in LVPs and I.V. sets: Automated microscopic and Coulter Counter methods, *Pharm. Tech.*, *2*, 31 (1978).

61. W. H. Coulter, U. S. Patent 2,656,508, 1953.

62. Coulter Electronics, Inc., *Theory of the Coulter Counter*, Bulletin T-1, 1958.

63. R. Cartmel and H. N. Gerrard, The Coulter Counter, *Pharm. J.*, *191*, 383 (1963).

64. O. Q. Ulbrich, *Size Analysis of Fine Particles and Results Obtained with an Electrical Sensing Zone Particle Analyzer*, Paper presented before Instrument Society of American Conference, New York, Sept. 26, 1960.

65. S. M. Blaug and R. E. Sarabia, Determination of particulate matter in intravenous solutions using the Coulter Counter, *Bull. Parenter. Drug Assoc.*, *29*, 74 (1975).

66. H. G. Schroeder and P. O. DeLuca, Theoretical aspects of particulate matter monitoring by microscopic and instrumental methods, *J. Parenter. Drug Assoc.*, *34*, 183 (1980).

67. M. J. Groves and J. F. G. Major, Assessment of particulate material in normal saline solution, for injection B.P. by means of the Coulter Counter, *Pharm. J.*, *193*, 227 (1964).

68. R. W. Lines, An insertable orifice tube for *in situ* contamination counts of solutions in opened ampoules and vials using the Coulter Counter, *J. Pharm. Pharmacol.*, *19*, 701 (1967).

69. M. J. Groves, Coulter Counter estimation of particles retained on terminal filtration units, *Pharm. J.*, *208*, 550 (1972).

70. T. G. Somerville and M. Gibson, Particulate contamination in ampuls, *Pharm. J.*, *211*, 128 (1973).

71. A. B. Bikhazi, J. A. Shiatis, and A. F. Haddad, Quantitative estimation of particulate matter in pharmaceutical preparations intended for intravenous administration, *J. Pharm. Sci.*, *66*, 181 (1977).

72. R. J. Lantz, E. G. Shami, and L. Lachman, Application of the HIAC particle counter to monitoring particulate matter in parenteral solutions I: A preliminary study, *Bull. Parenter. Drug Assoc.*, *30*, 234 (1976).

73. P. J. Davies and J. D. Smart, Evaluation of the Royko 367 small-volume sample feeder for estimation of particulate contamination in ampoules, *J. Pharm. Pharmacol.*, *31*, 108P (1979).

74. G. H. Hopkins and R. W. Young, Correlation of microscopic with instrumental particle counts, *Bull. Parenter. Drug Assoc.*, *28*, 15 (1974).

75. T. Rebagay, H. G. Schroeder, and P. P. DeLuca, Particulate matter monitoring II: Correlation of microscopic and automatic counting methods, *Bull. Parenter. Drug Assoc.*, *31*, 150 (1977).

76. Y. S. Lim, S. Turco, and N. M. Davis, Particulate matter in SVPs as determined by two methods, *Amer. J. Hosp. Pharm.*, *30*, 518 (1973).

77. J. Blanchard, J. A. Schwartz, D. M. Byrne, and D. B. Marx, Comparison of two methods for obtaining size distribution characteristics of particulate matter in large-volume parenterals, *J. Pharm. Sci.*, *67*, 340 (1978).

78. L. Ernerot, Particle counting in infusion fluids, *Acta Pharm. Suec.*, *11*, 1 (1974).

79. R. J. Whitlow, T. E. Needham, and L. A. Luzzi, Generation of particulate matter in large-volume parenteral containers, *J. Pharm. Sci.*, *63*, 1610 (1974).

4
Package Integrity Testing

INTRODUCTION

The assurance that freedom from sterility, pyrogens, and particulates is maintained in parenteral products depends to a significant degree on the integrity of the packaging system designed to protect the product throughout its shelf-life. The inability of a packaging system to prevent the ingress of microbial and particulate contamination is a most serious deficiency. Various package integrity tests are available to assure the reliability of the container/closure system in preventing contamination.

A search of the literature reveals a dearth of information related to package integrity testing. In part, this must be due to (a) a relative lack of defective parenteral package seal problems, and (b) the inherent difficulty in testing the integrity of all parenteral packaging systems except for the leaker testing of glass-sealed ampuls.

Basically, five types of packaging systems exist for parenteral products:

1. Ampuls
2. Vials
3. Bottles (glass and plastic)
4. Plastic bags
5. Cartridges and syringes

All of these package systems contain single-dose products except for vials. Vials use a rubber stopper as a seal which can reseal itself following puncture by a needle. Multiple-dose vials contain an antimicrobial preservative agent intended to protect the product against accidental contamination. Products intended for single dose generally do not contain an antimicrobial agent. Thus, if microorganisms are able to enter the product due to a lack of package integrity, no internal protection exists against such incursion.

The United States Pharmacopeia (1) states that "containers are closed by fusion, or by application of suitable closures, in such a manner as to prevent contamination or loss of contents." However, no statement exists pertaining to the testing necessary to evaluate the integrity of the container/closure system in their ability to prevent contamination or loss of contents.

Leaker testing traditionally is linked to the detection of leaks in flame-sealed glass ampuls. Other parenteral container/closure systems usually are not subjected to end-product leaker testing. The main reason for this is the belief that container/closure interfaces cannot withstand the high vacuum or high pressure used in primary leaker test methods. However, various methods do exist for testing the seal integrity of vials and bottles, including the use of vacuum and pressure.

TYPES OF PROBLEMS IN PARENTERAL PACKAGE INTEGRITY

Package integrity is compromised any time the drug product contained in the package system becomes inadvertently exposed to outside conditions. Gross lack of package integrity, e.g., a tear or hole in a plastic container, a visible crack in a glass container, or a visible opening between a rubber closure and its normal resting position, can be detected rather easily. The inner contents have either leaked or spilled out, or detectable changes in color or clarity have occurred. The real hazards of package integrity defects arise when such defects are unnoticed by even the most observant human inspector or state-of-the-art testing methods. The phenomenon of glass ampul microfractures represents an excellent example of a package integrity problem that easily can, and usually does, escape human and physical test detection. Crouthamel (2) presented valid evidence that the common dye vacuum leaker test for ampuls cannot detect areas of devitrification on the tips of ampul containers. When ampul tips are sealed, the smooth morphology of normal vitreous glass will change to a crystalline state,

a process called devitrification. Crouthamel cited the research of
one American ampul manufacturer claiming that up to 3% of all ampuls undergo devitrification in a small area of the ampul tip during
sealing. The significance of this change is that within the area of
devitrification, at any time after sealing, a fracture of the crystalline glass may occur. Scanning electron photomicrographs show
the widths of the fractures to vary from 0.15 to 0.5 μm, with some
extending to 2.5 μm. The lower limit for capillary size detection
with the dye bath test is 3 μm. Various studies, as reviewed by
Crouthamel, have reported ampuls showing dried material on their
tips with no visible penetration of the dye (3—6). Since the dye
bath test cannot detect fractures caused by devitrification because
of the extremely small size of the fracture, the parenteral industry
must realize that the potential for contamination exists with a small
percentage of each ampul lot tested for leakage by the vacuum dye
test.

LEAKER TESTS FOR AMPULS

Ampuls are flame-sealed by one of two methods: tip sealing or pull
sealing. Tip sealing (Figure 4.1) involves melting glass at the tip
of the neck of a rotating ampul to the point where the ampul opening is hermetically closed. Pull sealing (Figure 4.2) involves heating the neck of the ampul below the tip and, once the glass begins
to melt, using forceps manually or automatically to pull the ampul
tip away from the rotating ampul body.

Ampul leakers develop as a result of slight errors in the sealing
process. Pull seals are less prone to error than tip seals because
the pulling action and subsequent rotation completely close the capillary tube formed during sealing. Tip sealing introduces two potential causes of inadequate sealing. If the tip is heated excessively, a bubble of glass will form. The wall of the glass bubble
will be very thin and fragile and can easily be broken. On the
other hand, if the tip is heated insufficiently, a pinhole will remain,
thus producing the leaker. While pinholes are more likely to result
from inadequate tip sealing, pull sealing also can cause leakers if
the rotating action following the tip being pulled away is inadequate.

Numerous methods for detecting ampul leakers have been used
(see Table 4.1). However, the most widely used method continues
to be the vacuum dye method or modification thereof. The electronic pinhole-detection system has gained significant acceptance
in recent years as a faster and more sensitive detector of ampul
leakers.

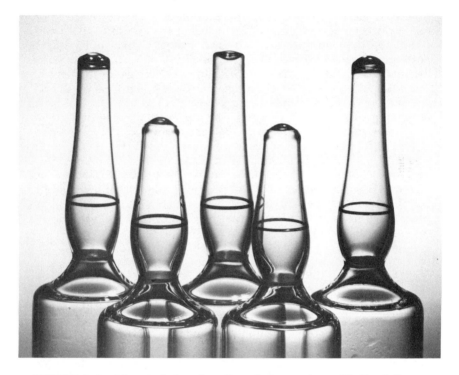

FIGURE 4.1 Tip-sealed and pull-sealed ampuls, with the taller ampuls being tip-sealed. (Courtesy of Cozzoli Machine Co., Plainfield, New Jersey.)

Vacuum Dye Leaker Test

The basic procedure involves placing sealed ampuls in a dye bath, applying vacuum for a certain time period or periods, removing and rinsing the ampuls, and visually inspecting for the presence of dye inside the ampul. An example of a standard operating procedure for ampul leaker testing by the vacuum dye method may be seen in Table 4.2.

Various dyestuffs have been used in leaker testing. Characteristics of an ideal dyestuff are listed in Table 4.3. The most commonly used dyes are blue dyes, such as methylene blue (0.1–1.0%), FDA Blue No. 1 (20%), and FDA Blue No. 2 (2%). Other dyes that are available for leaker testing include D and C Red No. 19 (0.1%), guinea green (5%), and fluorescein (2%). Green to yellow-green

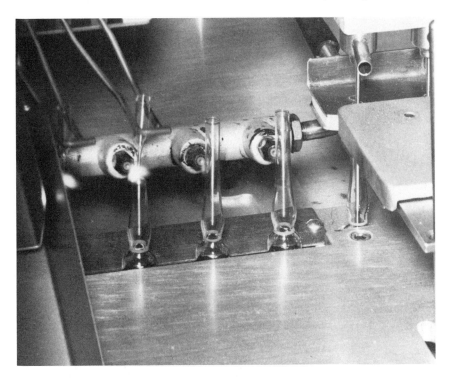

FIGURE 4.2   Ampuls being pull-sealed on a Cozzoli Model FPS 2
ampul-filling and -sealing machine.   (Courtesy of Cozzoli Machine
Co., Plainfield, New Jersey.)

dyes are most sensitive to the human eye while blue, violet, and
red dyes are the colors least sensitive to human eye detection.
Red and yellow dyes are employed infrequently and cannot be applied to amber ampuls.   Fluorescents have not been suitable in
leaker tests (7).

The purpose of the vacuum period(s) is to create an artificial
pressure differential across the sealed opening of the ampul or
other container.   Any seal defect will allow dye to enter the container because of differences in pressure between the inside and
outside of the conatiner.

As itemized in Table 4.2, ampuls are rinsed in a detergent solution followed by purified water before being transferred to the dye
tank.   Ampuls may remain upright when immersed in the dye solution if they are hot, e.g., in leaker testing immediately after the

TABLE 4.1 Leaker Tests for
Ampul Container Systems

---

1. Visual
2. Vacuum dye
3. Pressure dye
4. Autoclave dye
5. Dry port bubble
6. Dye after autoclaving
7. Microbial broth immersion
8. Fluorescein penetration
9. Helium—high frequency
10. Electrical discharge
11. Ultrasonics
12. Radionuclides

---

autoclave cycle. Otherwise, cold ampuls should be immersed with
the tips down. This will maximize the pressure differential exerted
at the ampul tip during the leaker test.

Vacuum cycles vary depending on the size of ampul, size of load,
size of testing chamber, and experience of the manufacturer. The
most common vacuum cycle consists of one vacuum cycle with 25—28
inches of mercury pulled for a minimum of 15 minutes. Some experts advocate the application of multiple vacuum pulls for short
periods (5—10 minutes) of time.

Various factors (see Table 4.4) affect the visibility of the dye
should it gain entrance into a defective ampul. Obviously, color
may be detected more easily in colorless ampuls compared to amber
containers. Agitation of a leaker ampul with dye concentrated at
the tip will permit dilution of the dye in the product solution and
limit or deny detection of the faulty ampul. Amber ampuls will
accentuate this problem. Even some colorless ampuls with a bluish
tinge will mask a diluted and weakly light-absorbing blue dye.
Dyes used in leaker testing are weak organic acids and bases whose
color and color intensity depend on solution pH. Ampul products
possessing solution pHs beyond the pH range of maximum color
type and intensity of the dye will neutralize the color or reduce
the degree of color discrimination. For example, meperidine hydrochloride, in the presence of light, will neutralize the color of methylene blue entering the pinhole of a faulty ampul. Color stability
of organic dyes is affected by reducing and oxidizing agents and
surface active agents. If the time interval between the dye test

TABLE 4.2   Typical Procedure for Leaker Testing by the
Vacuum-Dye Method

---

1. After autoclaving, the ampuls are rinsed in a detergent solu-
    tion to remove medicament (from broken ampuls) from the
    outer surface of the ampuls.

2. Ampuls are then rinsed in purified water to remove detergent
    solution.

3. Racks of ampuls are transferred to a dye tank that contains
    150 ml of Colorbot Blue 1 dye solution per 500 liters of
    Purified Water. The formula of the Colorbot Blue 1 used is:

Sodium CMC[a]	10.0 g
F D and C Blue No. 1	200.0 g
Alcohol SD No. 20[a]	3.0 ml
Chloroform [a]	3.0 ml
Purified water q.s. to	1000.0 ml

4. Racks of ampuls are submerged in the dye solution and a
    vacuum of 25–28 inches of mercury is applied for a minimum
    of 15 minutes.

5. Vacuum is neutralized rapidly using "quick release" valves.

6. Ampuls remain submerged in dye solution for a minimum of 15
    minutes after vacuum neutralization.

7. Racks are removed from dye tank and are rinsed several times
    (in successive tanks of purified water) to remove dye solution
    from exterior surface of ampuls.

---

[a]The Sodium CMC, alcohol, and chloroform serve no purpose as
far as the leaker test is concerned. They are incidental ingredients in the stock dye solution used for the leaker test.

TABLE 4.3   Attributes of Dye for Testing

---

1. Low order of toxicity
2. Dye approved for drug use
3. Chemically and physically color-stable over broad pH range
4. Non-interactive with contents of ampuls
5. High intensity of color
6. Solubility in a cleaning solvent
7. Insensitive to light and heat
8. Easily disposed to meet EPA requirements

TABLE 4.4 Factors Affecting Visibility of Dye in Ampuls

---

1. Extinction coefficient of the dye

2. Wavelength at which dye maximally absorbs light

3. Oxidation-reduction potential of the dye

4. Viscosity, color, and pH of the ampul contents

5. Product formulation components, e.g., anti-oxidants, surfactants

6. Color of the ampul glass

7. Size of the ampuls

8. Time interval between the dye test and the visual inspection

9. Degree of agitation of ampuls following the dye test

10. Capability of the inspector

---

and inspection for leakers is too long, dye entering a faulty ampul containing these agents will degrade and lose its color.

During leaker testing by the dye vacuum test, there exists the possibility that the dye solution will contaminate the contents of the ampul. To minimize this possibility, the dye solution should be prepared from a sterile concentrate and diluted with sterile water immediately before use. Dye solution may be used more than once if it is stored at 80°C.

Removing dye from the outside of the container following leaker testing can be a major problem. The more concentrated the dye, the more difficult it becomes to rinse it away completely. In some instances, a surfactant (e.g., Polysorbate 80) may be added to the dye solution to aid in the removal process.

The amount of dye solution entering a circular pore depends on Poiseuille's Law (8):

$$t = \frac{8 \times \ell \times V \times n}{\pi \times r^4 \times \Delta P}$$

where t is the minimum time required for a volume V of dye solution of viscosity n to penetrate a capillary of length ℓ and radius r when the pressure differential is ΔP. According to Poiseuille's equation, the amount of dye solution entering the pore is directly proportional to ΔP and t, and inversely proportional to n. McVean et al. (5) calculated that for 1-ml glass ampuls having a pore opening (r) of 0.1 μm and a wall thickness (l) of 3.8×10^{-2} cm, immersed into a 1% methylene blue solution of viscosity 10^{-2} poise and a pressure differential applied of 2×10^{6} dynes-cm^{-2} (2 atm), the time necessary for perceptible (10^{-5} ml) dye solution penetration would be approximately 2200 hours:

$$t = \frac{8 \times 3.8 \times 10^{-2} \times 10^{-5} \times 10^{-2}}{3.14 \times (0.05 \times 10^{-4})^{4} \times 2 \times 10^{6}} \times \frac{1}{3600} = 2200 \text{ hours}$$

Reducing the time of the vacuum cycle to 0.5 hours, the test procedure according to Poiseuille's equation would detect ampuls having an opening of approximately 0.8 μm diameter.

Helium-Spark Method

This method was first described by Stafficker in 1956 (3). It is still in use but is not a common leaker test method.

Prior to the flame sealing of ampuls, air is displaced by an inert gas such as helium. The sealed ampuls having helium in the airspace are placed in a vacuum chamber and vacuum applied for 30 minutes. Following vacuum, a high-frequency spark coil is brought next to the ampuls, one at a time. If a pinhole is present, the charge can enter the ampul. A reaction occurs with the helium gas, resulting in a discharge that is blue. If there is no pinhole, there will be no discharge. The minimum pinhole size detectable by the helium-spark method is claimed to be 7 μm, compared to 14 μm detectable by the dye test (3).

Electronic Detection of Pinholes

The Nikka Densok company of Japan developed a high-frequency spark test system to detect automatically the presence of pinholes in ampul products of various sizes. Ampuls are conveyed into a detecting unit (Figure 4.3) and exposed to a high-frequency voltage. The presence of a pinhole permits the discharge current to enter the ampul. The current inside the container will be detected by the system and subsequently rejected from the conveyer.

The principle of successful operation of the high-frequency spark test system involves an electrically conductive solution contained

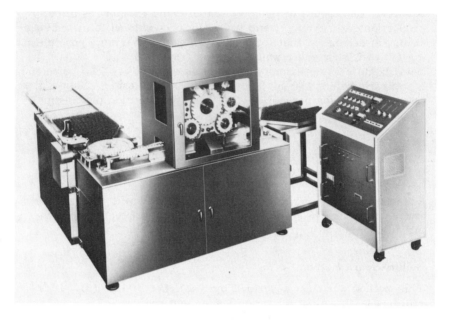

FIGURE 4.3   The Nikka-Densok HDA-11 Pinhole Inspector Machine
with the detecting unit in the center.   (Courtesy of Seidenader
Equipment, Inc., Morristown, New Jersey.)

within a non-conductive container. Without a defect on or in the
glass ampul, the electric spark cannot be maintained and the ampul
will not register a signal alerting the system to reject it.

Several advantages are claimed for the high-frequency spark
system over other leaker test systems. These are listed in Table
4.5. Major advantages include the detection of extremely small pinholes (the minimum size claimed is 0.5 μm); continuous, non-human
inspection; application to amber-colored containers; and the speed
of inspection (18,000 ampuls per hour).

Broth Immersion Leaker Test

Leaker tests are supposed to determine the capability of the con-
tainer/closure system to prevent microbial contamination of the
container contents. A direct method of testing this capability is
through the use of the broth immersion leaker test.

The bath solution in this test is a microbial broth containing a
known concentration of suspended microbial cells cultured from a

TABLE 4.5 Advantages of Automatic Pinhole Detection by the
Nikka-Densok System

---

1. *Higher inspection accuracy.* The system can detect extremely
   small pinholes that have been undetectable by any conventional tests such as the dye testing method. Thus, it is most
   suitable for preventive countermeasures for secondary contamination which might be caused by bacteria.

2. *Higher processing speed.* The system can be operated at a
   speed as high as 18,000 ampuls per hour.

3. *No fear of contaminating solution inside ampul.* Because of
   an electrical detecting method, the system is a clean unit, and
   thus, unlike the dye testing method, this system offers no
   danger of contaminating the solution inside an ampul.

4. *Applicable to colored ampuls and colored solution.* Because
   inspection is conducted not visually but electrically, the system performance is not affected by colored ampuls and colored
   solution.

5. *Simple handling and safety operation.* All an operator has to
   do is depress buttons; no particular training for operating
   the unit is necessary. Several safety devices are incorporated.

6. *Easier part removal.* At the time of cleaning or size part
   change, parts such as starwheels, screws, etc. can easily be
   removed and mounted without the use of tools.

7. *Easier coupling with preceding and following stages.* With a
   feeding conveyor used as an accumulator, the unit can immediately be coupled with the preceding stage. The employment
   of starwheels on both feeding and discharging devices enables
   the unit to be easily incorporated in line.

---

single species. Preparation of an inoculum for the microbial challenge test is described in Table 4.6. Ampuls are placed in a vacuum dessicator containing the broth inoculum. Vacuum is drawn
for 10–15 minutes at 25–30 mm. Following the vacuum cycle, the
dessicator is transferred to an incubator set at 30–35°C. After
incubation for two weeks, the ampuls are disinfected by adding
10 ml clorox to each liter of medium and allowing a 10-minute exposure period. The ampuls then are inspected for growth as evi-
denced by the presence of a cloudy or turbid solution.

TABLE 4.6   Preparation of Inoculum for Microbial Challenge Test

---

1. Maintain *Pseudomonas diminuta* on nutrient agar slants (incubate 18—24 hours at 30°—35°C). Use ATCC #19146.

2. Streak a nutrient agar plant from a fresh slant and incubate 48 hours at 30°—35°C. *P. diminuta* will appear as small (1—2 mm) circular, slightly convex, colonies with an entire edge. Color is a very light tan. Perform Gramstain (very small gram-negative rods).

3. Select a well-isolated colony and inoculate 10—20 ml Tryptic Soy Broth in a 50-ml flask containing a spin bar (length 1 inch). Incubate on a magnetic stirrer at approximately 60 rpm for 24 hours at 30°—35°C, or employ another proven method.

4. Inoculate 2 ml of the above spin culture into one liter of Saline Lactose Medium[a] for the test.

5. Perform plate counts at 0 time from the inoculated Saline Lactose Medium to confirm concentration of *P. diminuta* (10^6 per ml) minimum.

---

[a]1.   Dissolve 7.6 g ACS sodium chloride in 970 distilled water.
2.   Dissolve 1.3 g dehydrated Lactose Broth (BBL) in 100 ml distilled water.
3.   Add 30 ml of the Lactose Broth solution to 970 ml of the sodium chloride solution.
4.   Autoclave at 121°C for 15 minutes or per approved autoclave cycle.

This type of microbial challenge is described as a dynamic immersion challenge. It is a severe test and has obvious disadvantages, such as the time and expense required for conducting the test and the risks involved in using microbial challenge media. A major application of broth immersion testing is to check or validate the adequacy of the dye vacuum/pressure leaker test.

Radionuclide Leaker Test

This test, described by DeLuca and his co-workers (9, 10), employs a short-lived radioactive substance such as Technetium 99m or Chromium 51, included in a solution with or without a dye. Ampuls are immersed in the solution, and pressure and/or vacuum applied. They are then decontaminated and dried to remove the radionuclide on the outside of the container. If the test solution contained a dye, the ampuls are inspected for the presence of color inside the container. Ampuls passing the color inspection are then tested by scintillation counting for the presence of radioactivity. If a maximum permissible radiation count is exceeded, the ampul is rejected.

Radionuclide leaker tests overcome some major limitations of the conventional dye leaker tests. Dye leaker tests are dependent upon dye entering the defective ampul, the color of dye being easily discernable by the human inspector, and the solution pH of the ampul product not causing a neutralization of the color of the dye. In the results of Butler et al. (9), 10.2% of the ampuls tested failed to produce discernable color while containing excessive amounts of Technetium 99m.

On the other hand, radionuclide leaker tests are very time-consuming and require protection from exposure to radiolabeled materials. The amounts of radioactivity used, 10 millicuries of Tc 99m and 5 millicuries of Cr 51, are low doses of low energy gamma emitters, yet must be handled with every safety precaution. Time consumption increases not as a result of the leaker test itself, but in the preparation and calibration of the gamma counter and because of the need for blanks to correct for the natural disintegration of the radionuclide during the test.

LEAKER TESTS FOR PARENTERAL CONTAINERS OTHER THAN AMPULS

Final package leaker tests for non-ampul parenteral products are seriously limited by the nature of the package system and its vulnerability to high vacuum or pressure forces. Vials, glass bottles, and cartridges have rubber closures or plunger tips which cannot withstand the range of pressure/vacuum extremes employed in conventional dye leaker tests. Plastic containers also cannot withstand high vacuum or pressure. Thus, alternative approaches have been used to determine container/closure integrity in lieu of leaker tests used for glass ampuls.

Vials

Vials depend on a rubber closure to seal the vial opening and protect the vial contents from contamination entering through that opening. The integrity of this container/closure interface is, therefore, of extreme importance in guaranteeing the sterility and stability of the inner contents. Various approaches have been utilized to determine the integrity of the container/closure seal. These have been summarized in the Parenteral Drug Association *Technical Information Bulletin No. 4* (11).

Vacuum Retention

This method does not test the final product. Rather, it is designed to evaluate the ability of a rubber closure to maintain a vacuum. Following the evacuation of the headspace of a vial, the closure is pushed firmly into the neck of the vial, thereby establishing a sealed container. The vacuum retained over a period of time or following a long (60 minute) autoclave cycle is then determined using a modified vacuum gauge puncturing the rubber closure.

Vacuum Chamber

Containers, after filling, stoppering, and sterilization, are placed in a vacuum chamber in an inverted position. Vacuum is applied for a certain period of time, then released, and the containers are inspected for leakage. A common alternative method utilizing the vacuum chamber involves filling the containers with a dye solution, proceeding as above, and determining package integrity by noting the transmission, if any, of dye from the inner contents to the outside of the container.

Internal Pressure

This method is similar to the vacuum retention method except that pressure rather than vacuum is used to create an artificial pressure differential at the closure/container interface. Internal pressure is achieved by filling under pressure or by generating internal pressure after filling by hot air immersion, hot water immersion, or autoclaving. Containers are subsequently evaluated by observating for encrustation at the closure seal point, loss of internal pressure, or leakage of contents through the seal.

Seal Force Test

The West Company produces an instrument called the Seal Force Tester, which will measure the tightness of vial closures (12). The device measures the residual compressive force in the rubber stopper after sealing with an aluminum seal. The tester is shown in Figure 4.4. As can be seen, the tester is manually operated and consists basically of a force gauge, cap anvil, bottle rest, and microscope.

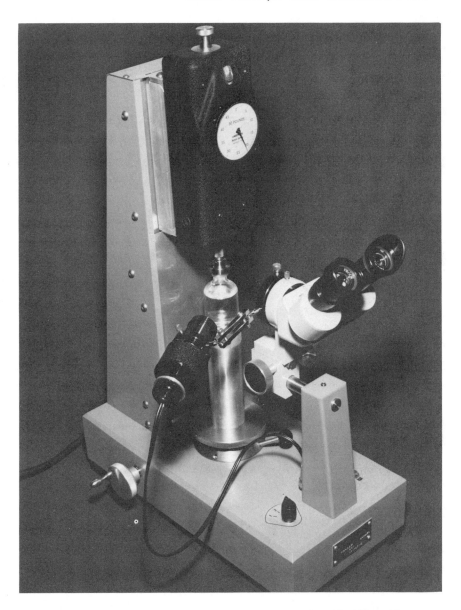

FIGURE 4.4   The West Seal Force Tester, Model WG-005. (Courtesy
of the West Company, Phoenixville, Pennsylvania.)

A sealed vial is placed and adjusted on the bottle rest for proper viewing of the vial cap through the microscope. The mechanical force gauge is manually pressed down on the top of the closure with the cap anvil. When the compressional force of this operation just exceeds the residual compressive force in the rubber closure, the aluminum cap will begin to move downward. The human operator will detect this first downward movement through the 20 × microscope, stop applying additional force, and read the force in pounds of pressure applied. The process is repeated twice using other positions on the closure. The three force readings are averaged and compared to a reference force experimentally determined to be an acceptable force level for a tight seal for the particular vial closure system.

The tester can be used to measure seal tightness for any conventional closure, including three-piece tear-off seal and Flip-off caps. The tester, however, cannot detect a leak in a seal that is due to a void or defect in the glass or rubber.

Recently, the West Company developed a fully automated instrument called the Seal Force Monitor (13) (Figure 4.5). The device not only measures compressional force of the closure at the cap, but also can determine the total force required to crimp a cap onto a vial.

During the capping operation, a force transducer measures the varying forces applied on the closure. Electrical signals from the transducer are sent to a microprocessor within the instrument. The microprocessor stores in its memory signals from good vials, producing a reference profile. All subsequent vials are compared electronically to the reference profile. Containers not conforming to this predetermined set of acceptable force measurements are automatically rejected. Defects detected and rejected by the Monitor include missing caps, missing stoppers or liners, broken glass, defective glass finishes, and vials requiring excessively high or low capping forces.

Microbiological Challenge

Vials are filled with culture media, usually trypticase soy broth, then sealed with the particular rubber closure. Media-filled containers are then challenged microbiologically using one or more of the following four approaches (11).

1. Static--aerosol challenge: Expose sealed containers to periodic challenge by generating aerosol containing the challenge organism.

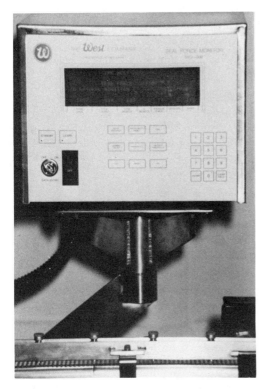

FIGURE 4.5   The West Seal Force Monitor, Model WG-008.
(Courtesy of the West Company, Phoenixville, Pennsylvania.)

2. Static--immersion challenge: Expose sealed containers to
    periodic challenge by immersing in a suspension of challenge
    organisms.
3. Static--ambient challenge: Expose sealed containers to am-
    bient conditions and monitor periodically for evidence of
    microbial growth.
4. Dynamic--immersion challenge: Expose sealed containers to
    periodic challenge by immersing in a suspension of challenge
    organisms, with simultaneous additional stress of pressure/
    vacuum if warranted by the normal conditions of product
    storage.

An application of the integrity testing of vial closure systems
was published recently by scientists of the Upjohn Company (14).

Two methods were used to evaluate the adequacy of vial closure systems representing a variety of vial neck sizes, closure formulations, and product types. One method involved suspending the vials in an inverted position for two hours at room temperature followed for four hours at 49 ± 3°C (15) and then observing the vials for evidence of leakage. The other method used a microbiological challenge test like the static-ambient challenge test described above. Additionally, some of the culture media-filled vials were inverted during the storage period (up to 48 months) to permit the medium to contact the container/closure interface. Then, at yearly intervals, these inverted vials were tested by the static-immersion challenge method described above using *Escherichia coli* (10^8 colony forming units/ml) as the microbial challenge. The results of these tests are given in Table 4.7. The authors concluded that these integrity tests were superior to the sterility test for evaluating container/closure integrity for the following reasons:

1. The tests are based on conclusive physical and microbiological evaluations.
2. They simulate actual product handling and storage conditions.
3. Quantitative data on contamination rates are provided.
4. The integrity of the container/closure system is rigidly challenged.

However, it must be noted that because there were no failures in any of the vials on either the physical or microbiological evaluations, one must question the validity of these methods to detect any lack of container/closure integrity. Such "positive" controls probably should have been tested along with all the marketed product samples evaluated in this published study.

Bottles (Large-Volume Parenterals)

All of the tests described for vial container/closure integrity evaluation can be applied to large-volume bottles. In addition, two methods have been used: the spark-coil method and the water hammer test.

Spark-Coil Method

This method is used for vacuum-sealed bottles. A high-frequency spark coil brought near an individual bottle will generate a blue spark in the headspace of the bottle interior if a vacuum is present. If no vacuum is present, indicative of a faulty seal, either a purple spark or no spark at all will be seen.

TABLE 4.7 Microbial Growth and Growth Promotion Results in Representative Vial Closure Systems

Vial neck diameter (mm)	Stopper formulation	No. units put on test	Test interval completed (months)	No. units showing growth	Growth promotion results[a]
9	Natural rubber-W	490	48	0	+
13	Natural rubber-WA	390	48	0	+
	Natural rubber-TA	500	36	0	+
	Bromobutyl rubber	500	24	0	+
	Natural rubber-T	500	36	0	+
	Butyl rubber-T	500	36	0	+
	Natural rubber-TM	500	24	0	+
	Butyl rubber	500	24	0	+
20	Natural rubber-W	500	24	0	+
	Bromobutyl rubber-W	500	24	0	+
	Butyl rubber-TA	500	24	0	+
	Butyl rubber-T	500	36	0	+
	Natural rubber-WM	432	48	0	+
	Bromobutyl rubber-WM	500	24	0	+
	Butyl rubber-TM	500	36	0	+
30	Natural rubber-W	462	48	0	+
TOTAL	16	7774		0	

[a] + indicates a satisfactory growth promotion test for each of the four test organisms after the longest test interval completed.
Source: Ref. 14.

Water Hammer Test

Although a crude test, the water hammer test has some application as a spot-check seal integrity test during the bottle-manufacturing process and as a simple quality assurance test in hospital practice. A bottle is selected off the assembly line following the generation of a vacuum and sealing of a rubber closure. The bottle is inverted and a rubber hammer is used to stroke the bottom surface of the bottle. A high-pitched, distinctive cracking sound will indicate the presence of a vacuum inside the bottle. This, in turn, indicates the sound integrity of the seal at the bottle-stopper interface.

Large-Volume Plastic Containers

These containers are among the most difficult to evaluate for leakers or seal integrity. Two very basic test procedures are (a) observing for fluid leakage in the external pouch after autoclaving the container, and (b) applying pressure (hand or mechanical) to the bag and observing for any leakage of the inner contents.

Package integrity of plastic bags can be ascertained microbiologically by employing the same procedures as was described in the section on vials.

REFERENCES

1. United States Pharmacopeia, 21st edition, Mack Publishing, Easton, Pennsylvania, 1985, p. 1138.
2. T. G. Crouthamel, Microfractures in parenteral glass ampuls, *J. Parenter. Sci. Tech.*, *35*, 18 (1981).
3. C. F. Stafficker, Leaker detection by helium, *Bull. Parenter. Drug Assoc.*, *10*, 10 (1956).
4. W. J. Artz, W. T. Gloor, Jr., and D. R. Reese, Study of various methods for detecting leaks in hermetically-sealed ampuls, *J. Pharm. Sci.*, *50*, 258 (1961).
5. D. E. McVean, P. A. Tureck, G. L. Christenson, and J. T. Carstensen, Inadequacies in leakage test procedures for flame-sealed ampuls, *J. Pharm. Sci.*, *61*, 1609 (1972).
6. I. G. Brizell and J. Shatwell, Methods of detecting leaks in glass ampuls, *Pharm. J.*, *21*, 73 (1973).
7. *Reliability in Checking Ampoules for Leaks*, National Social Welfare Board, Stockholm, Sweden, April, 1968, p. 3.
8. A. N. Martin, J. Swarbrick, and A. Cammarata, *Physical Pharmacy*, 2nd edition, Lea & Febiger, Philadelphia, Pennsylvania, 1969, p. 508.

9. L. D. Butler, J. J. Coupal, and P. P. DeLuca, The detection of ampul leakers using short-lived radionuclides, *J. Parenter. Drug Assoc.*, *32*, 2 (1978).
10. U. S. Patent No. 4,267,499.
11. *Technical Information Bulletin No. 4*, Parenteral Drug Association, Inc., 1983.
12. *WG-005 Seal Force Tester Bulletin No. 676*, The West Company, Phoenixville, Pennsylvania.
13. J. T. Connor, In-process verification of closure seal integrity, *J. Parenter. Sci. Tech.*, *37*, 14 (1983).
14. W. R. Frieben, R. J. Folck, and A. Devisser, Integrity testing of vial closure systems used for parenteral products, *J. Parenter. Sci. Tech.*, *36*, 112–116 (1982).
15. Federal Specifications, PP-C-186C, *Containers, Packaging and Packing for Drugs, Chemicals, and Pharmaceuticals*, November 19, 1976, Defense Personnel Support Center, Directorate of Medical Material, Philadelphia, Pennsylvania.

appendix I

APPENDIX I   Example of Standard Operating Procedure for Sterility Testing by Direct Inoculation*

Purpose: To describe the USP test procedure for sterility testing by direct inoculation.

Equipment and Supplies

1. Soybean casein direct (SCD) medium, trypticase soy broth (TSB) medium—sterile test tubes of appropriate size, one for each sample plus three controls
2. Fluid thioglycollate medium (FTM)—sterile test tubes of appropriate size, one for each sample plus three controls
3. Sterile syringes or pipets, one for each sample
4. One incubator at 32°C
5. One incubator at room temperature
6. Laminar flow (LF) workbench
7. Sterile Tyvek gown
8. Sterile disposable cap
9. Sterile mask
10. 70% Alcohol
11. Betadine or pHisohex
12. Urethane wipes

Procedure

Steps	Comments
1. The operator shall wear a sterile coat, mask, and disposable cap. The operator shall wash hands thoroughly with a disinfectant scrub before donning sterile gloves.	
2. Wipe inside, top, and counter surfaces of LF workbench with suitable surface disinfectant.	Take care to avoid splashing surface of HEPA filter. Surface disinfectant is usually 70% alcohol but others may be used and should be from time to time.

*Reprinted by permission of Dr. K. E. Avis, College of Pharmacy, University of Tennessee, Memphis, Tennessee.

APPENDIX I   (continued)

Steps	Comments
3. Wipe all exposed surfaces of vials, ampuls, tubes of culture media, and other containers with surface disinfectant before placing them in LF workbench.	
4. All sterile items having an outer wrapping should have the wrapping removed at the edge of the LF workbench and the sterile inner item introduced aseptically into the workbench.	Alternatively, the outer wrapping may be wiped with a disinfectant prior to placing in the workbench, but this is less desirable.
5. After all supply items have been introduced into the LF workbench, the operator should change to a new pair of sterile gloves or, preferably, partner will then perform the critical aseptic steps using uncontaminated gloves.	The usual hand disinfectant is pHisohex or Betadine. Sterile latex or PVC gloves may be worn but are not required.
6. For vials, remove protective seal and disinfect exposed rubber closure with alcohol wipe.	Leave damp, but there should be *no* pool of disinfectant.
7. For ampuls, break neck at score mark, pointing toward side of workbench rather than HEPA filter.	Avoid splattering of HEPA filter with liquids. Do not place hands between filtered air source and critical site.
8. Use a sterile syringe or pipet to transfer the appropriate volume of product to each test tube containing either sterile TSB or FTM.	Refer to USP sterility test procedures for appropriate volumes of media and product inocula.

APPENDIX I   (continued)

Steps	Comments
9. After all required product samples have been inoculated, inoculate one additional tube of TSB and FTM with product. Then inoculate each tube with a loopful of standard test organism culture of a spore strip.	These tubes will serve as positive controls to show that the test organism grows in the presence of the product.
10. Two additional tubes of SCD and FTM should be used as controls. One tube of each medium should be inoculated with loopful of test organism and the other tube left uninoculated.	The inoculated tubes will show that the culture media support growth of microorganisms and the blank tubes will confirm the sterility of the culture media.
11. Incubate the samples at appropriate temperatures and observe after 3, 7, and 10 days for presence of microbial growth.	Incubate FTM at 32°C and TSB at 25°C [room temperature (RT)]. Longer incubation may be required at times to permit slow growers to develop.
12. Record results on quality control record sheet.	
13. Sterilize used culture media and clean tubes after incubation.	

appendix II

APPENDIX II   Example of Standard Operating Procedure for
Sterility Testing by Membrane Filtration*

Purpose: To describe a method for the use of membrane filters
in the sterility testing of sterile products.

Equipment and Supplies

1. Sterility sterility test filter holder unit—Millipore Sterifil,
   Falcon unit
2. Membrane filter, 0.45 μm, 47 mm, hydrophobic edge
3. Sterile needles, syringes, or administration sets—20
4. Sterile trypticase soy broth (TSB), 100 ml tubes—3
5. Sterile fluid thioglycollate medium (FTM), 100 ml tubes—3
6. Sterile diluting fluid, 100 ml—3
7. Sterile scissors
8. Sterile forceps, smooth tip, 4½–6 in. stainless steel
9. Sterile disposable gloves
10. Alcohol, 70% denatured
11. Urethane wipes
12. Laminar flow hood (LFH)
13. Blue plastic base with hole for Falcon unit
14. Test samples
15. Sterile gown, cap, and mask

Procedure

Steps	Comments
1. The operator shall wear a sterile coat, mask and disposable cap. The operator shall wash hands thoroughly with a disinfectant scrub before donning sterile gloves.	
2. Wipe inside, top, and counter surfaces of LF workbench with suitable surface disinfectant.	Take care to avoid splashing surface of HEPA filter. Surface disinfectant is usually 70% alcohol but others may be

---

*Reprinted by permission of Dr. K. E. Avis, College of Pharmacy, University of Tennessee, Memphis, Tennessee.

APPENDIX II   (continued)

Steps	Comments
	used and should be from time to time.
3. Wipe all exposed surfaces of vials, ampuls, tubes of culture media, and other containers with surface disinfectant before placing them in LF workbench.	
4. All sterile items having an outer wrapping should have the wrapping removed at the edge of the LF workbench and the sterile inner item introduced aseptically into the workbench.	Alternatively, the outer wrapping may be wiped with a disinfectant prior to placing in the workbench, but this is less desirable.
5. After all supply items have been introduced into the LF workbench, the operator should change to a new pair of sterile gloves or, preferably, partner will then perform the critical aseptic steps using uncontaminated gloves.	The usual hand disinfectant is pHisohex or Betadine. Sterile latex or PVC gloves may be worn but are not required.
6. Remove overseals from the necks of test samples, previously disinfected ampuls, multidose vials or large-volume containers. Wipe the rubber diaphragm or neck of ampuls with 70% alcohol.	Do not leave excess alcohol on closure.
7. For ampuls, break neck at score mark, pointing toward side of workbench rather than HEPA filter.	Avoid splattering of HEPA filter with liquids. Do not place hands between filtered air source and critical site.

APPENDIX II   (continued)

Steps	Comments
8. Attach previously sterilized filter unit to vacuum source. Filter unit should contain 47 mm, 0.45 µm hydrophobic edge membrane.	Use rubber tubing. Make certain a trap flask is used to collect filtrate overflow. Falcon units may be stabilized by setting in hold of blue plastic base.
9. Transfer the prescribed volume from sample to upper chamber of filter unit. (a) Use a needle and syringe to withdraw the prescribed inoculum of product from ampuls or vials. Insert needle through rubber closure of vials or into opened ampuls and withdraw prescribed sample for test, or (b) use a needle and transfer set to transfer the prescribed volume of solution from large volume containers. Insert spike of set through rubber diaphragm.	See USP sterility test for number of samples and inoculum size. One syringe may be used for all samples since the samples will be pooled, but a new sterile needle should be used for each vial or bottle.
10. Wipe injection diaphragm of filter unit with 70% alcohol.	
11. Insert needle of syringe or transfer set through previously asepticized diaphragm or administration set.	Use proper aseptic technique. Be sure critical sites are bathed directly in LF air. A closed system is essential to prevent drawing environmental contaminants into upper chamber of filter unit.
12. Inject from syringe or apply vacuum to transfer	Avoid direct injection on membrane as it may puncture the

APPENDIX II (continued)

Steps	Comments
prescribed volume of solution to be tested into upper chamber of the filter.	filter. Preferably inject down side or into liquid layer above filter.
13. Apply vacuum to pull, or prime to push solution through filter.	Pull or push all solution through filter.
14. Repeat steps 6–10 until all units have been tested.	
15. When all solution has been filtered, turn off vacuum and carefully remove top.	Turn off vacuum carefully to avoid reverse surge. Care must be taken to avoid accidental contamination.
16. Aseptically pour 100 ml of sterile diluting fluid down internal sides of chamber and onto the filter. Replace top, apply vacuum, and filter the fluid.	To remove residual portions of product, rinse all surfaces efficiently.
17. Repeat step 13 two more times.	
18. After all solution has been filtered, turn off vacuum and carefully remove top half of filter assembly.	Exercise caution to avoid contamination.
19. Using sterile forceps and scissors, remove membrane from holder and cut into two halves.	Hold filter and cut over a sterile surface so that the membrane will not be accidently contaminated if it falls.
20. Place one half of the membrane in a sterile tube of SCD, the other half in a tube of FTM, and incubate at prescribed temperatures for the specified time.	Use sterile forceps to place filter in culture media tubes. See USP for incubation times and temperatures.

APPENDIX II   (continued)

Steps	Comments
21. Include a positive and a negative control tube of each medium.	Innoculate one tube of each medium with a loopful of spore suspension or a paper strip of *B. subtilis* as a positive control, plain medium as a negative control.
22. Incubate the samples at appropriate temperatures and observe after three and seven days for presence of microbial growth.	Incubate FTM at 32°C and TSB TSB at 25°C (RT). Longer incubation may be required at times to permit slow growers to develop (e.g., 10–14 days).
23. Thoroughly wash all equipment used. Make certain to empty and clean vacuum trap flask.	This is to remove residual product and media.
24. Return used equipment to proper locations.	
25. At the end of incubation period observe samples for growth and record results of tests on appropriate report forms.	
26. Sterilize used culture media and clean tubes after incubation.	

appendix III

APPENDIX III   Example of Methods Used to Clean, Assemble,
Sterilize, and Make Final Connections with Membrane Filtration
Equipment

Cleaning

1. Mainfold: After testing has been completed for the day,
   flush completely with hot water followed by distilled water,
   then drain thoroughly and allow to dry overnight.

2. Filter holders: Clean after each use by using a mechanical
   dishwasher with an extended five-minute wash cycle or by
   immersing in a detergent solution.   After a soaking period
   in the detergent solution, rinse in hot tap water and distilled water, backflushing the fritted-glass bases to dislodge any trapped material.   Parts may be wiped dry with
   ling-free toweling.   If holders are to be sterilized the same
   day, dry the fritted-glass base with lab air or vacuum.

3. Swinney Adapter: After use, soak in alcohol, detergent,
   or other suitable agent.   Disassemble and remove used prefilters from wire screen, dry, and reassemble with clean
   prefilters.

Assembly

1. Slide a rubber stopper over the outlet tube of each filter
   holder base and place each base in its manifold support.
   Place a funnel on each base and clamp in place with a spring-
   action clamp.

2. Insert a host adapter into each rubber funnel cover and
   attach a three-way stopcock to the adapter.   A similar
   adapter in the end of the rubber tubing at each manifold
   position is attached to the opposite end of the three-way
   stopcock.

3. On the side arm of the stopcock, place a Swinney Hypodermic Adapter containing a single 13-mm diameter Microfiber Glass Prefilter.

4. Place two 13-mm diameter Microfiber Glass Prefilters in each
   of the remaining six Swinney Hypodermic Adapters and
   attach each adapter to its fitting on the side of the manifold
   valves.

5. Wrap the ends of the manifold openings with paper for
   sterilization.

APPENDIX III   (continued)

Sterilization

1. Open all manifold stopcocks. Failure to open stopcocks may result in damage to the filters and inadequate sterilization. Residual moisture could also damage the filters. Steam sterilize the entire assembly.

Final Connection

1. When the assembly is cool, move it to a sterile area and close all stopcocks. Connect the vacuum tubing to a large receiver (water trap) beneath the bench and connect the receiver to a vacuum source.

2. Flame and connect flushing manifold to a pressurized source of sterile diluting fluid.

3. Aseptically place a sterile membrane filter onto each of the filter funnel units on the sterility test unit. The apparatus is now ready to use.

4. Extra filter funnel units, with membrane filters in place, may be wrapped individually and autoclaved. These can be put in place on the sterility test unit and used for testing after the original units have been used.

appendix IV

APPENDIX IV   Aseptic Procedures at the Laminar Flow
Workbench*

Note: The laminar flow workbench with HEPA filtered air, when
functioning properly, provides a Class 100 clean environment
suitable for aseptic procedures. However, the procedures utilized must take advantage of the functional features of the LF
workbench in order not to compromise the achievements possible
therein.

1. The LF workbench should be located in a buffer area that
    is clean and orderly, thereby enhancing the functional effi-
    ciency of the workbench.

2. At the beginning of each workday and each shift, and when
    spillage occurs, the workbench surface should be wiped
    thoroughly with a clean, non-linting sponge dampened with
    distilled water. The entire inside of the workbench should
    then be wiped with another clean, non-linting sponge damp-
    ened with a suitable disinfectant, such as 70% alcohol.

3. The blower should be operated continuously. However,
    should there be a long period of non-use, the blower may
    be turned off and the opening covered with a plastic cur-
    tain or other shield. The blower then should be operated
    for at least 30 minutes and all the internal surfaces of the
    hood should be cleaned thoroughly and wiped with a dis-
    infectant before use.

4. Traffic in the area of the workbench should be minimized
    and controlled. The workbench should be shielded from
    air currents that might overcome the air curtain and carry
    contaminants into the work area.

5. Supplies entering the buffer area should be isolated in a
    remote place until they can be decontaminated by removing
    outer packaging. That is, outer cartons and packaging
    materials should not be brought near the workbench. All
    supply items should be examined for defects prior to being
    introduced into the aseptic work area.

---

*Reprinted by permission of Dr. K. E. Avis, College of Phar-
macy, University of Tennessee, Memphis, Tennessee.

APPENDIX IV   (continued)

6. Supplies to be utilized in the workbench should be decon-
    taminated by wiping the outer surface with 70% alcohol, or
    other suitable surface disinfectants, or by removing an
    outer wrap at the edge of the workbench as the item is
    introduced into the aseptic work area.

7. If the workbench is located in a non-aseptic area, such as
    a hospital pharmacy, before approaching the workbench,
    personnel must thoroughly scrub hands and arms with a
    detergent followed by an appropriate skin antiseptic. Each
    must then don a clean cap that provides complete coverage
    of head hair and a clean, non-linting, long-sleeved coat
    with elastic or snaps at the wrist and, preferably, a solid
    front panel. A face mask must be worn if there is no
    transparent barrier panel between the operator's face and
    the aseptic work area or if the operator has facial hair or
    an upper respiratory condition that promotes sneezing and
    coughing.

8. After proper introduction of supply items into the aseptic
    workbench, they are to be arranged in a manner such that
    operations can take full advantage of the direction of lam-
    inar air flow, that is, either vertical or horizontal. Supply
    items within the workbench should be limited in order to
    minimize clutter of the work area and provide adequate
    space for critical operations. A clean pate of HEPA fil-
    tered air must be provided directly from the filter source
    to the critical work site. No supplies and no movement of
    the personnel should interpose a non-sterile item or sur-
    face between the source of the clean air and the critical
    work site. Therefore, no objects should be placed hori-
    zontally behind the critical work site or above the critical
    work site in a vertical laminar flow workbench. Also, all
    work should be performed at least six inches within the
    workbench to avoid drawing contamination in from the
    outside.

9. All supply items should be arranged so that the work flow
    will provide maximum efficiency and order.

10. It should be noted that the hands are clean but not sterile.
    Therefore, all procedures should be performed in a manner
    to minimize the risk of touch contamination. For example,

APPENDIX IV   (continued)

---

the outside barrel of a syringe may be touched with the hands since it does not contact the solution, but the plunger or needle should not be touched.

11. All rubber stoppers of vials and bottles and the neck of ampuls should be cleaned, preferably with 70% alcohol and a non-linting sponge, prior to the introduction of the needle for removal or addition of drugs.

12. Avoid the spraying of solutions on the workbench screen and filter.

13. After every admixture, the contents of the container must be thoroughly mixed and should then be inspected for the presence of particulate matter or evidence of an incompatibility.

14. Filtration of solutions to remove particulate matter is frequently necessary, particularly when admixtures have been prepared. A small volume of solution may be filtered by attaching an appropriate membrane filter to the end of a syringe, using the plunger to force the liquid through the filter. Note: To avoid rupture of the membrane, force may be applied in one direction only through the filter. Where larger volumes of solutions must be filtered, this may be accomplished by means of an appropriate in-line filter and an evacuated container to draw the solution through the filter or, preferably, by means of a pressure tank of nitrogen, or other inert gas, to apply pressure to the liquid in the container to force it through the in-line filter. In the latter situation, the pressure must be maintained low enough to avoid the risk of explosion of the solution container (usually a maximum of 10−12 p.s.i.g.). There are at least two disadvantages of the vacuum system as compared with the pressure system: (a) any leakage draws contamination into the container and system; (b) the vacuum may be lost, thereby stopping the procedure.

15. The porosity of the appropriate membrane filter is determined by the objective of the filtration. To remove particulate matter, a 1 μm porosity filter should be satisfactory. To sterilize a solution, a 0.2 μm filter would be required.

APPENDIX IV   (continued)

16. The completed preparation should be provided with an appropriate tamper-proof cap or closure to assure the user that the integrity of the container has been maintained until the time of use.

17. The workbench should be cleaned with a clean sponge, wet with distilled water, as often as necessary during the workday and at the close of the workday. This should be followed by wiping the area with a sponge with an appropriate disinfectant.

18. During procedures, used syringes, bottles, vials, and other supplies should be removed, but with a minimum of exit and re-entry into the workbench.

appendix V

APPENDIX V   Comparison of Published Limulus Amebocyte Lysate (LAL) Methods, Including the Four Basic Methods (Gel-Clot, Turbidimetric, Colorimetric, and Chromogenic) and Their Modifications*

Method	Reagents needed	Equipment needed	Endpoint
Gel-Clot (1, 2)	LAL	37°C water or dry bath	Gel-Clot
Turbidimetric (3, 4)	LAL	37°C water or dry bath or oven and spectrophotometer	Turbidity
Colorimetric (5)	LAL and Lowry protein reagent	37°C water or dry bath or oven, spectrophotometer, and centrifuge	Blue
Chromogenic (6, 7)	LAL, acid, and chromogenic reagent buffer	37°C water or dry bath or oven and spectrophotometer	Yellow
Nephelometric (8)	LAL	37°C water of dry bath or oven and nephelometer	Turbidity
Kinetic (9, 10)	LAL	Abbott MS-2	Turbidity
Kinetic (11)	LAL	Modified microplate reader	Turbidity
Slide (gel-clot) (12, 13)	LAL	37°C oven and microscope slide	Gel-clot
Slide (dry-up) (14)	LAL	37°C oven and microscope slide	Dry-clot
Slide (wells) (15)	LAL, dye, and petrolatum	37°C oven and microscope slide	Gel-clot

*Reproduced in part from T. J. Novitsky, *Med. Dev. Diagn. Ind.*, Jan. 1984.

Incubation time (min)	Skill level	Sensitivity (EU/ml)	Cost per test (in $)	Total operator time (min)
60	Low	0.02—1.0	0.45—4.00	60
30—60	Moderate to high	0.01—1.0	0.90—2.00	60
10—20	High	0.05—0.5	0.96—4.50	60
10—20	High	0.05—0.5	0.96—4.50	60
30—60	Moderate to high	0.01—1.0	0.90—2.00	60
20—90	Low	0.0005—500	4.00	20
20—90	High	0.0005—500	0.45—4.00	60
30—45	Moderate	0.02—1.0	0.05—0.40	60
30	Moderate	0.5—2.5	0.05—0.40	60
30	Moderate	0.15—1.0	0.05—0.40	75

APPENDIX V   (continued)

Method	Reagents needed	Equipment needed	Endpoint
Slide (capillary) (16)	LAL	37°C oven, micro- scope slide, and capillary tube	Gel-clot
Slide (stain) (17)	LAL and dye	37°C oven and microscope slide	Gel-clot
Slide (phase contrast) (17)	LAL	37°C oven, micro- scope slide, and microscope	Gel-clot
Micromethod (18)	LAL and dye	37°C oven and microplate	Gel-clot
Microtechnique (19)	LAL	37°C oven tube of dye, and capillary tube	Gel-clot
Microdilution (20)	LAL and dye	37°C oven and microplate	Gel-clot
LAL-bead (21)	LAL	37°C water or dry bath, beads, tray, and rocker platform	Gel-clot
Radioisotope (22)	LAL and 125- labeled coagulogen	37°C water or dry bath, centrifuge, and gamma counter	Gel-clot
Rocket (23)	LAL and anti- coagulogen antibody	37°C water or dry bath and gel electrophoresis	Gel-clot

Incubation time (min)	Skill level	Sensitivity (EU/ml)	Cost per test (in %)	Total operator time (min)
30—45	Moderate	0.02—1.0	0.05—0.40	60
30	Moderate	5.0	0.05—0.40	60
30—45	Moderate	0.02—1.0	0.05—0.40	75
75	Moderate	0.50—1.0	0.09—0.80	60
45	Moderate	0.05—1.0	0.05—0.40	75
60	Moderate	0.30—1.0	0.25—2.00	60
90	Moderate to high	5.0	0.45—4.00	90
40—50	High	0.05—0.6	2.00—5.00	120
60	High	0.05	2.00—5.00	180

REFERENCES TO APPENDIX V

1. J. F. Cooper, J. Levin, and H. N. Wagner, Jr., Quantitative comparison of *in vitro* and *in vivo* methods for the detection of endotoxin, *J. Lab. Clin. Med.*, *78*, 138–148 (1971).

2. J. H. Jorgensen and R. F. Smith, Rapid detection of contaminated intravenous fluids using the Limulus *in vitro* endotoxin assay, *Appl. Microbiol.*, *26*, 521–524 (1973).

3. J. D. Teller and K. M. Kelly, A turbidimetric limulus amebocyte assay for the quantitative determination of gram negative bacteria, *Biomedical Applications of the Horseshoe Crab (Limulidae)* (E. Cohen, Ed.), Alan R. Liss, New York, 1979, pp. 423–433.

4. B. R. Albaugh and C. B. Chandler, Automated methodology for the Limulus amebocyte lysate (LAL) assay using the Multiskan Microplate Reader, *Endotoxins and Their Detection with the Limulus Lysate Test* (S. Watson, J. Levin, and T. Novitsky, Eds.), Alan R. Liss, New York, 1982, pp. 183–194.

5. R. Nandan and D. R. Brown, An improved *in vitro* pyrogen test: To detect picograms of endotoxin contamination in intravenous fluids using Limulus ameobocyte lysate, *J. Lab. Clin. Med.*, *89*, 910–918 (1977).

6. T. Harada, T. Morita, S. Iwanaga, et al., A new chromogenic substrate method for assay of bacterial endotoxins using Limulus hemocyte lysate, *Biomedical Applications of the Horseshoe Crab (Limulidae)* (E. Cohen, Ed.), Alan R. Liss, New York, 1979, pp. 209–220.

7. Y. Fujita and C. Nakahara, Preparation and application of a new endotoxin determination kit, Pyrodick, using a chromogenic substrate, *Endotoxins and Their Detection with the Limulus Lysate Test* (S. Watson, J. Levin, and T. Novitsky, Eds.), Alan R. Liss, New York, 1982, pp. 173–182.

8. J. A. Dubczak, R. Cotter, and R. F. Dastoli, Quantitative detection of endotoxin by nephelometry, *Biomedical Applications of the Horseshoe Crab (Limulidae)* (E. Cohen, Ed.), Alan R. Liss, New York, 1979, pp. 403–414.

9. T. J. Novitsky, S. S. Ryther, M. J. Case et al., Automated LAL testing of parenteral drugs in the Abbott MS-2, *J. Parenter. Sci. Technol.*, *36*, 11–16 (1982).

10. J. H. Jorgensen and A. S. Reichler, Automation of Limulus amoebocyte lysate pyrogen testing, *J. Parenter. Sci. Technol.*, *36*, 96–98 (1982).

11. V. B. Ditter, K. P. Becker, R. Urbaschek et al., Detection of endotoxin in blood and other specimens by evaluation of photometrically registered LAL-reaction-kinetics in microtiter plates, *Prog. Clin. Biol. Res.*, *93*, 383–392 (1982).

12. P. Frauch, Slide test as a micro-method of a modified Limulus endotoxin test, *J. Pharm. Sci.*, *63*, 808–809 (1974).

13. H. Goto, M. Watanabe, and S. Nakamura, Studies on a simple Limulus test, a slide method, *Jpn. J. Exp. Med.*, *47*, 523–524 (1977).

14. H. Goto and S. Nakamura, Dry up method as a revised Limulus test with a new technique for gelation inhibitor removing, *Jpn. J. Exp. Med.*, *49*, 19–25 (1979).

15. K. L. Melvaer and D. Fystro, Modification micromethod of the Limulus amebocyte lysate assay for endotoxin, *Appl. Environ. Microbiol.*, *43*, 493–494 (1982).

16. D. J. Flowers, A microtechnique for endotoxin assay by using Limulus lysate, *Med. Lab. Sci.*, *36*, 171–176 (1979).

17. S. Okuguchi, Improvement of the micromethod for the Limulus lysate test, *Microbiol. Immunol*, *22*, 113–121 (1978).

18. J. G. Kreeftenberg, H. G. Loggen, J. D. Van Ramshorst et al., The Limulus amebocyte lysate test micromethod and application in the control of sera and vaccines, *Dev. Biol. Standard*, *34*, 15–20 (1977).

19. A. Gardi and G. R. Arpagaus, Improved microtechnique for endotoxin assay by the Limulus amebocyte lysate test, *Anal. Biochem.*, *109*, 382–385 (1980).

20. R. B. Prior and V. A. Spagna, Adaptation of a microdilution procedure to the Limulus lysate assay for endotoxin, *J. Clin. Microbiol.*, *10*, 394–395 (1979).

21. N. S. Harris and R. Feinstein, The LAL-bead assay for endotoxin, *Biomedical Applications of the Horseshoe Crab (Limulidae)* (E. Cohen, Ed.), Alan R. Liss, New York, 1979, pp. 265–274.

22. R. S. Munford, Quantitative Limulus lysate assay for endotoxin activity: Aggragation of radioiodinated coagulogen monomers, *Anal. Biochem.*, *91*, 509–515 (1978).

23. L. Baek, New, sensitive rocket immunoelectrophoretic assay for measurement of the reaction between endotoxin and Limulus amoebocyte lysate, *J. Clin. Microbiol.*, *17*, 1013–1020 (1983).

Index